Dennis Wong

Joe Mah
Dec. 2, 2017

YIN YANG QI
The Art of Balancing Health

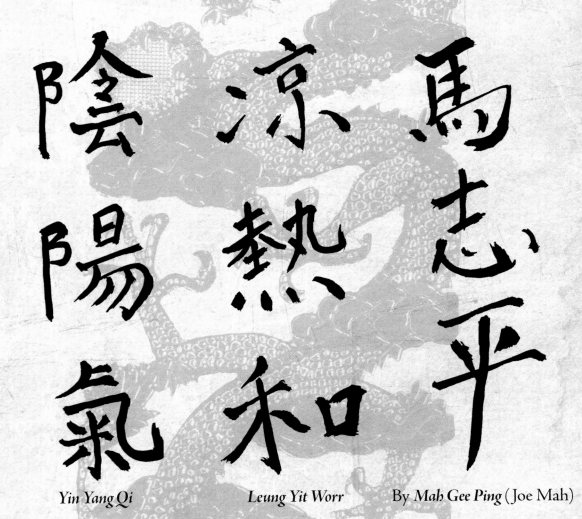

陰　涼　馬

陽　熱　志

氣　和　平

Yin Yang Qi　　　*Leung Yit Worr*　　　By *Mah Gee Ping* (Joe Mah)

Website:
yinyangqi.com

First Edition 2010
Published by Hubstar International Inc.,
Montreal, Quebec, Canada.

Photo credits: Jonathan Blair-Joly of Multi-Graf Inc., LaSalle, Quebec, Canada.
Artistic Designer: Norman Quon - Montreal, Quebec, Canada.

Printed in Canada by Transcontinental Printing

Preface

About This Book

This book is about Chinese wellness concepts and related food therapy that keep the body in appropriate balance. These techniques are used to enhance health, promote fitness and slow the aging process. It presents the ancient Chinese concepts of maintaining bodily equilibrium through the use of appropriate foods, primarily special soups. It discusses these complex, oriental concepts in a simple manner that can be grasped by anyone. In so doing, it touches on bodily, mental and spiritual health; and on how these can be maintained and enhanced through moderation, a proper diet and physical balance. This book is based on the following Chinese concepts:

• There is a basic balance in nature and all phenomena can be reduced to an interaction between two opposing forces. This is the Yin-Yang principle that was conceptualized more than 5,000 years ago.

• Traditional Chinese medicine has transferred the Yin-Yang concept to the human body. For wellness, there must also be a balance among bodily forces that is achieved by adopting a lifestyle of moderation, proper diet and appropriate actions. When applied to the human body this concept is known as *leung-yit*.

• Every human body is different and has its own balance of *leung* ("coolness" related to Yin) and *yit* ("hotness" related to Yang). Everyone must develop a personal understanding of an appropriate bodily balance.

• *Leung-yit* imbalance is a principle cause of illness. Prevention of illness by following a proper diet that maintains bodily balance is the key to good health. When combined with moderation and an appropriate lifestyle, maintaining proper balance also slows the aging process.

• The body is constantly using jing/essences. There are two sources of jing/essences: from what we eat (food, drink, vitamins and supplements) and from essences already stored within the body. If we supply the body with an appropriate diet, it will not have to extract any jing/essences from within itself.

• Premature depletion of stored jing/essence may cause the body to fatigue and age prematurely. Soups, fruits, vegetables, beans and herbs have various health benefits that the Chinese include in their diet to maintain a jing/essence balance. A food may have health benefits (*yow yick*) when it contains jing/essences required by the body.

• The Western influence upon Chinese commerce, culture, cuisine and thinking is undeniable. But what can the West learn from China? The most valuable thing that can be learned is how to live a long and healthy life, without depending on medicines.

• Permitting the body to deplete its internal supply of jing/essence is damaging and causes premature aging. The lost internal jing/essence can never be fully recovered. An appropriate diet is needed to prevent premature depletion of internal jing/essence. For centuries the Chinese have used long boiled soups to extract important essences from various herbs, plants and seeds. Many of these recipes are contained in this book.

• Also vital in maintaining good health is moisturizing. This concept is more than just drinking fluids to keep hydrated. It consists of using moisturizing essences to create internal moisture that heals. This is called *yuen fay* meaning deep moisturizing of the lungs. Skilled Chinese herbal experts have long used moisturizing to maintain good health. This book emphasizes healing by drinking moisturizing soups and juices.

• Maintaining good health lies in understanding what your body is telling you; recognizing the symptoms of imbalance and the need for certain essences. It also includes discontinuing specific foods or practices that cause problems and consuming special foods, especially soups that bring the body back into balance.

• The Chinese diet emphasizes eating dark green vegetables which contain large amounts of chlorophyll. This book contains a Chinese vegetable section with cooking instructions.

• No Chinese meal is complete without Chinese tea. This book discusses its importance in the overall diet.

This book contains recipes for over fifty traditional Chinese soups and congees, some tasty and some not so tasty, but all developed to address specific aspects of health and to maintain bodily balance. Some of these home-style soups are beneficial for preventing specific illnesses, while others provide a selection of special nutrients that are beneficial to general health. These soups are based on natural products such as herbs, mushrooms, seeds, nuts and vegetables that the Chinese have found beneficial in maintaining health and appropriate bodily balance. Some of these soups are cooked for more than four hours to extract the healing stock from the base ingredients. These soup recipes are balanced formulations that have been used for many generations and stand the test of time.

Acknowledgements

Writing this book has been a lifetime project which began when I was about four years old. I wish to thank my parents who had the foresight to encourage me to learn the secrets of how to stay young and healthy from various Chinese experts. I am thankful to the many herbal experts and scholars who taught me, especially George Young and Der Wing who spent years teaching me in their herbal stores. I am thankful to Wong Nan Moon for the guidance and positive influence he provided when I was young. I also want to thank Sam Wendel for encouraging me to write this book.

Having exposure to both the modern North American culture and the ancient Chinese culture has given me a unique perspective on the strengths and weaknesses of each and on how to combine these concepts for a common good. The ancient concepts that I mention in this book are easily understood by older ethnic Chinese but are not so easily understood by anyone else. Bridging the gap between these two distinct ways of thinking is no easy task. As I started writing this book, I began to realize that my expertise comes from many sources and that putting this knowledge into plain, concise, easily understood English would be a formidable task. So, I am thankful to Dr. Erling Nyborg for his assistance in putting it all together and his help in writing this book.

A special thanks to Norman Quon, who gave many useful comments on writing this book and who helped with the artwork and pictures. I am thankful to Linda Hackett for reviewing the text and encouraging me with her favorable comments. I thank Mark Ferrer for his help in editing the text. Most of all, I am thankful to my wife Jean for her love, understanding and support on this project.

Joe Mah, Montreal, October 2010

Disclaimer

The information and recipes contained in this book reflect the author's experience and do not intend to replace expert medical advice. There is no assurance that the reader will achieve any beneficial results from information contained this book. The information in this book is not intended as a substitute for any treatment that may have been prescribed by your doctor. Before making any changes to your diet, exercise regimen or way of life, consult your doctor to be sure that it is safe and appropriate for you.

No liability is assumed by the author, publisher, printer, distributor, reseller or anyone associated with this book with respect to the information or content of this book. They shall have neither responsibility nor liability whatsoever, to any person or business with respect to loss or damages caused or alleged to be caused, directly or indirectly by information contained in this book.

Notice

This book on oriental food therapy is not written by a medical doctor, a food scientist or a dietician. Instead, it is written by a second generation Canadian Chinese who learned the ancient teachings from the Chinese herbalists in Montreal's Chinatown and who has applied these teachings to his lifestyle for many years.

The food therapy of traditional Chinese medicine that has been passed on from generation to generation emphasizes maintaining good bodily health through:

- Appropriately balancing food intake and its bodily impact through wise application of the *Leung-Yit* (Yin Yang) principle.
- Maintaining regular sleeping habits and obtaining sufficient rest.
- Appropriate relaxation to clear the mind of its daily problems.
- Maintaining a fresh mental outlook that fosters positive thought.

This book makes no claims. The various soup recipes are listed as promoting individual health aspects. These listings are based on ancient teachings, many originating with those of the Yellow Emperor. They are not based on scientific evidence or fact. The reader must assess the benefits of the various recipes on his own. Possibilities such as allergies to various ingredients must also be considered. When in doubt consult your own doctor.

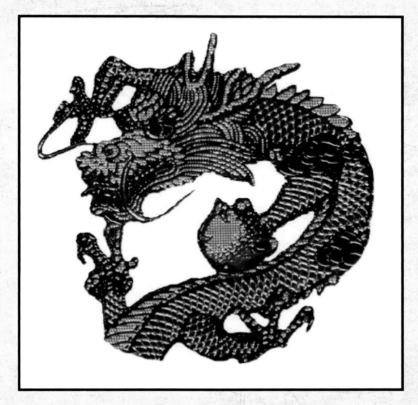

Those who know the Tao (the proper way of living) remain young, while those who do not know the Tao age prematurely.

Popular Chinese Belief

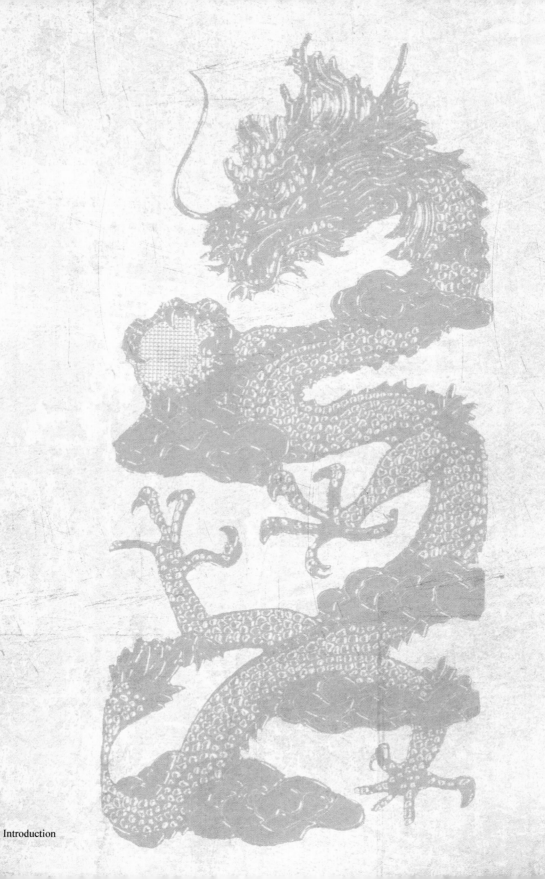

Introduction

Introduction

When I started writing this book on Chinese health concepts, I immediately came to realize that there is a major cultural gap between traditional Chinese medicine and Western medicine. Traditional Chinese medicine is normally proactive, while Western medicine is reactive. The Chinese method uses foods and soups to maintain an appropriate bodily balance to prevent illness and promote longevity; in the Western culture, we normally use medicines to cure illnesses after they have occurred.

Taoist Yin Yang Symbol

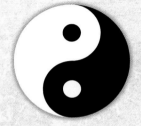

The title of this book, *Yin Yang Qi*, has a deep and significant meaning. According to Taoist legend, Yin and Yang came into being when the universe was created. At first there were only violently swirling gases, symbolized by two equal but opposite forces that formed swirling circles. In this early time, there was no solid matter and no life, but it contained the seeds of life. Although there was no solid substance, this stage is regarded as the mother of all things. That is why Taoists believe that formless (gas), forever swirling and emptiness is the foundation of everything. Over time, a third force- neutral came into being, solid matter began to form and life began. This third force was *Qi*, the breath of life. Life began with *Qi*; without *Qi* there could be no life.

Have *Qi*, have life.	No *Qi*, no life.
Have *Qi*, have hope	No *Qi*, no hope

Chinese proverb

Traditional Chinese medicine is based on an appropriate bodily balance of hot (*yit* or Yang) energies; cool (*leung* or Yin) energies and neutral (*worr*). This is done through *leung-yit* balancing of diet and the wise use of long boiled health soups. These soup recipes use hot, cool and neutral ingredients to promote balance.

One of the principal requirements for aging gracefully is control over bodily balance. When the body is out of balance, it reacts to regain balance. A knowledgeable person understands the imbalance and provides the nutrients that the body needs to bring it back into balance. Appropriately supplementing the body with what it needs prevents many health problems before they occur. This is the basic principle of traditional Chinese medicine.

It represents the three basic underlying concepts of traditional Chinese medicine, which date back over 5,000 years to the teachings of Huang Di, the Yellow Emperor[1] . Understanding and applying these concepts is the foundation of good health and longevity in traditional Chinese medicine.

When the Yin-Yang principle is applied to the human body it is known as the *leung-yit* concept. This is the basis of traditional Chinese medicine. For wellness, there must be a balance among bodily forces that is achieved by adopting a lifestyle of moderation, proper diet and appropriate actions. *Leung-yit* imbalance is a principle cause of illness. In this case, *leung* is characterized as "coolness" related to yin, while *yit* is characterized as "hotness" related to yang. This method is based upon how efficiently the body is able to resolve imbalances. When the body is no longer able to react, there is a breakdown of balance and life itself is in serious danger.

Qi (hay) is the breath or basic vital force that animates the human body. The body contains three principal energies; its internal energy, associated with Yin; its physical energy, associated with Yang and its animate energy, associated with *Qi*. The basic ingredients of the various health soups presented in this book have been selected to provide appropriate *leung or yit* to correct specific bodily imbalances and to maintain harmony among the three principal energies.

Balance and harmony are achieved by properly applying the Yin-Yang principle to lifestyle and to diet. Maintaining this balance and harmony leads to good health and longevity, while

[1 Numbers in superscript refer to the references listed on page 169]

imbalance among the three bodily energies sets the stage for chronic illness and premature aging. *Tao* signifies this way of combining the principles of Yin and Yang to maintain harmony with the natural order.

While this book refers to the teachings of Huang Di, it differs significantly from most books on traditional Chinese medicine. It does not follow the historical and theoretical approach taken by most traditional medical practitioners. Instead, it presents a layman's practical approach to the teachings of Huang Di, as initially learned as a student apprentice to herbalists George *"Young Guy Buck"* Young and Der Wing in their herbal stores in Montreal's Chinatown in the 1950's and 60's. It differs in an even more significant way in that the author is not a medical practitioner in traditional Chinese medicine but is instead a chartered accountant who has continued to practice what he learned as an apprentice, for the betterment of himself and his associates. This book has not been written by a professional expert but rather by a knowledgeable user trained in the practical applications of traditional Chinese food medicine.

This book presents the results of applying throughout life that which was learned at a young age from various Chinese experts. This continual practice turned the apprentice novice into a master in his own right. The health soup recipes contained in this book have been long used by the Chinese to restore bodily balance and harmony, as well as to slow the aging process. Many people regularly consume health soups as preventive measures against future ills; few know the exact purpose of each soup formulation. The author was fortunate in being taught by the experts to whom the Montreal Chinese came for advice. As a result this book not only provides a broad range of medicinal soup recipes, it also details the function and purpose of each formulation.

Health is the result of a balanced diet, proper exercise, mental strength and well being. Ill health results from the cumulative effects of disease, improper diet, lack of proper exercise and often poor mental attitude or spirit. Life's energy is sustained by air, water and food and influenced by our perception of life. When the energies are in balance health is enhanced. Problems begin with obstructed energy flow and imbalance. When the body is in balance, disease and illness are hard to develop; when the body is weak and out of balance, it is open to disease and illness. *Leung Yit* (Yin Yang) balance is viewed as the key to health and longevity, while imbalance is the route to bodily breakdown.

The way (*Tao*) to achieving good health and longevity is balance. A knowledgeable practitioner is able to monitor key bodily balances and remedy situations before problems develop. Remediation involves changing the diet, by reducing and removing offending items and replacing them with others that bring back bodily balance. Good health is the art of keeping the body in balance. It is not about a perfect diet or a perfect life-style; rather it is about keeping the body in tune and making various dietary adjustments to bring about balance, while taking everything in moderation.

Food is used as a medicine to prevent illness. Food and drink affect the internal bodily energy balance, cleansing and moisturizing. Long boiled health soups are used to promote health. Healthy eating means knowing what to eat, what not to eat, what food combinations are good and which are not.

In this book the author addresses four key elements for protecting the body from within through the appropriate use of health soups, teas and congees.

These include:

• Maintaining an appropriate *leung-yit* (cool-hot, Yin Yang) balance, both within the body and in the food being eaten.

• Drinking appropriate moisturizing soups, teas and fluids that prevent internal dryness and provide special nutrients for bodily healing and repair.

• Consuming special teas, soups and congees to maintain appropriate and regular cleansing of the digestive system, to break down fats and to remove impurities.

• Providing the body with the essential nutrients and essences that are needed for healing, rebuilding and maintaining bodily balance.

After reading this book you will be able to go into an authentic Chinese grocery store such as you find in many North American communities and order the ingredients needed to make a variety of traditional Chinese health soups – some deliciously tasty and some not so tasty but all developed to address specific aspects of the human body. You also will have learned the basic principles of Yin and Yang (*leung-yit*) and how to apply these principles towards building and maintaining a healthy body and living a long and productive life, while maintaining a young body and an admirable physique.

This is not another no-carbohydrate or no-fat diet book. It is rather a book about healthy living while doing everything in moderation. It is based on the wise teachings of the old Chinese masters as brought to North America by the first generations of Chinese immigrants. It is also based on an art still preserved in some parts of the Chinese community, but at risk of being lost or forgotten. In the last 100 years, much of these traditional skills and knowledge have been lost and forgotten. Newer generations have begun to disregard the old, believing that modern medicine has rendered these concepts and practices obsolete. This book is a cookbook, a health food book and an adventure in ancient Chinese culture all wrapped into one. Learn how to live a healthy, diet-free life by adopting the wisdom of the ancient Chinese.

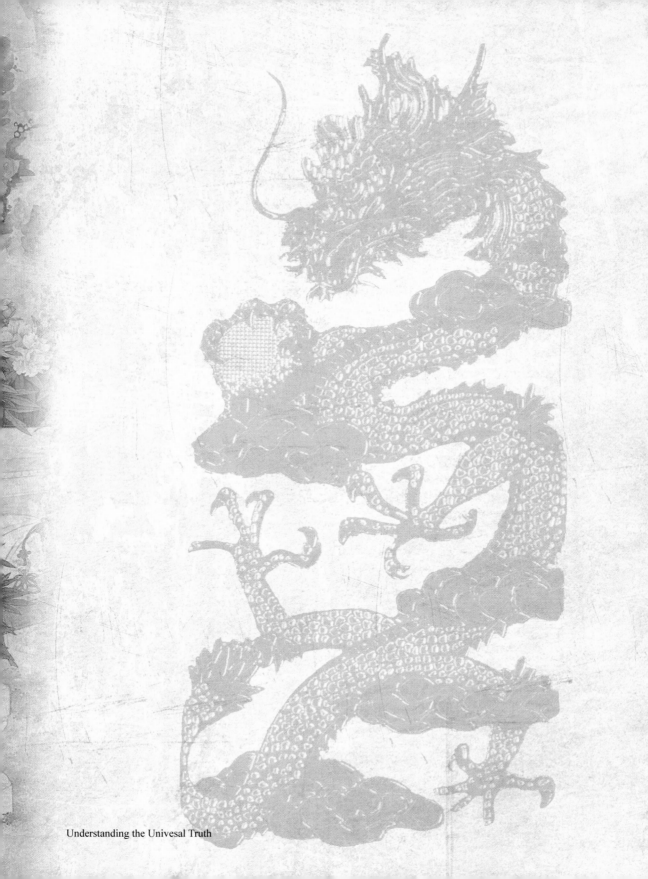

Understanding the Univesal Truth

Chapter 1

Understanding the Universal Truth

The Universal Truth

It was not until I began to write this book and took greater historical interest in the teachings of my ancestors that I realized that everything I had learned from my mentors in Chinatown was in reality based on the 5,000 year old teachings of the Yellow Emperor in traditional Chinese medicine. My mentors were really reinforcing that their understanding of how to maintain health and longevity was based on the Yellow Emperor's Universal Truth[2] . The following excerpts of Huang Di's discussions with his sages clearly illustrate these points:

During his reign, Huang Di discoursed on medicine, health, lifestyle, nutrition, and Taoist cosmology with his ministers Qi Bo, Lei Gong, and others. Their first discussion began with Huang Di inquiring, "I've heard that in the days of old everyone lived one hundred years without showing the usual signs of aging. In our time, however, people age prematurely, living only fifty years. Is this due to a change in the environment, or is it because people have lost the correct way of life?"

Qi Bo replied, "In the past, people practiced the Tao, the Way of Life. They understood the principle of balance, of yin and yang, as represented by the transformation of the energies of the universe. Thus, they formulated practices such as Dao-in, an exercise combining stretching, massaging, and breathing to promote energy flow, and meditation to help maintain and harmonize themselves with the universe. They ate a balanced diet at regular times, arose and retired at regular hours, avoided overstressing their bodies and minds, and refrained from overindulgence of all kinds. They maintained well-being of body and mind; thus, it is not surprising that they lived over one hundred years.

"These days, people have changed their way of life. They drink wine as though it were water,

indulge excessively in destructive activities, drain their jing—the body's essence that is stored in the kidneys—and deplete their qi. They do not know the secret of conserving their energy and vitality. Seeking emotional excitement and momentary pleasures, people disregard the natural rhythm and order of the universe. They fail to regulate their lifestyle and diet, and sleep improperly. So it is not surprising that they look old at fifty and die soon after.

Put more simply, my mentors stressed that those who live short lives often do not take care of their health. They fail to exercise caution in avoiding disease and contamination or simply never bother to learn what is healthy and what is not. Some develop unhealthy habits, such as smoking or excessive drinking. Others often ignore their health, placing greater importance on work, careers or pleasure. They follow an unhealthy lifestyle and simply don't care about their health until a major problem arises. Those who overwork and overstress themselves may wear down their bodies and their immune system opening the door to disease and illness. They also may allow their emotions to affect their minds and to harm their bodies.

Some simply have poor eating habits and don't balance their diets. They have irregular eating habits combined with the wrong types of food and don't know how to combine foods to achieve bodily balance. Others may lead destructive lifestyles. They may have bad sleeping habits that don't allow their bodies to rest and rejuvenate. They don't know how to conserve or rebuild their bodily energies. Since it is during sleep that the body is able to repair itself, having inadequate sleep can be very damaging. People who have short life spans often drain their protective jing/essence and deplete their *Qi* or life force.

Conversely, those who live long and healthy lives have mastered a working understanding of the Universal Truth. This they have done by caring for their bodies on an ongoing basis through:

- Understanding the principle of balance and staying centered by appropriately applying the Yin Yang principle.
- Knowing how to maintain bodily balance on an ongoing basis.
- Living in harmony with their environment and maintaining peace within themselves.
- Realizing the importance of maintaining external (physical or Yang), internal (supporting, sustaining or Yin) and *Qi* energies.
- Exercising.
- Eating a balanced diet.
- Knowing how to conserve their inherent (prenatal) jing/essence by consuming sufficient (postnatal) jing/essence in their diet.
- Keeping a regular schedule and avoiding overstressing their bodies and their minds.
- Practicing moderation and avoiding overindulgences.
- Having a positive attitude to life and living.

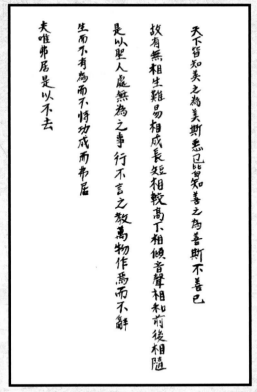

Under heaven all can see beauty as beauty only because there is ugliness[3] .

All can know good as good only because there is evil.

Therefore having and not having arise together.

Difficult and easy complement each other.

Long and short contrast each other;

High and low rest upon each other;

Voice and sound harmonize each other;

Front and back follow each other.

Maintaining an Appropriate Yin Yang Balance

The above verse from *Tao Te Ching*[3] describes Yin Yang well. Maintaining a Yin Yang balance is the central theme of all ancient Chinese teachings. Food and special health soups are used extensively to help the body regulate itself and to maintain its balance in equilibrium. Maintaining mental balance is also emphasized. Lopsided lifestyles are unbalanced because critical elements are missing. Traditionally, Chinese have strong family values and value their "face" or how they are perceived by their friends and community. Having a balanced lifestyle enables them to draw energy from their social circles and to maintain a purpose in life.

Maintaining an appropriate Yin Yang balance has a paramount influence on diet. At home, Chinese normally use cool cooking methods (steaming, boiling) and depend less upon hot cooking methods (deep frying, barbequing). Meat proportions are much smaller in traditional Chinese diets. There is less emphasis on meat and more emphasis on green vegetables, tofu, legumes, fish and seafood. Dairy product proportions are also much smaller than by North American standards. Home-style meals are far less greasy than restaurant fare.

Yin Yang implies that everything in the universe has an opposite. This means that anything can be counter balanced with its opposite. The traditional Chinese believe that chronic health problems develop due to imbalances. They pay close attention to what they eat and understand the importance of balance. They also look closely at the signs of imbalance and emerging health problems, such as dryness, skin tone, redness, pallor, breath smell, mental alertness and outlook. Major problems can be prevented by correcting small problems before they grow.

We drink cold drinks when we are hot and drink hot drinks to warm us up when we are cold. This is a simple example of Yin Yang balance. Traditional Chinese carry this concept to a much higher degree of sophistication. They adjust their diets in reaction to what is happening within their bodies. If there is a Yang (*yit* or hot) imbalance within the body the diet is adjusted by reducing or avoiding Yang (*yit* or hot) food and increasing the consumption of Yin (*leung* or cooling) food. There are several key Yin Yang concepts applicable to structuring balanced diets to maintain bodily health. These include:

• Assessing whether the overall bodily balance is in *leung or yit* (cold or hot, Yin or Yang). This measure is the the most important aspect for analyzing overall health and determining the type of imbalance.

• Moisturizing or drying.

• Speeding digestion or slowing digestion.

• Soothing or irritating.

• Cleansing or contaminating.

• Clearing or bloating.

• pH balance (acid or alkaline).

• Ascending or descending body heat (fever or chills).

• Strengthening or weakening.

Traditional Chinese medicine recognizes a direct correlation between what is happening within our bodies and what we are eating. The opposites listed above not only reflect a possible bodily imbalance, they also reflect the properties of specific food ingredients that can overcome each imbalance. The specific properties of various food ingredients and the overall healing properties of Chinese health soups are discussed in detail in the following chapters.

Food combinations have a direct impact upon wellness and upon the Yin Yang balance. Eating healthy healing food is important. You must be proactive to maintain an appropriate Yin Yang balance. Health is an ongoing challenge and should be addressed daily. An appropriate strategy is to constantly vary the diet to address potential imbalances or simply to serve as a preventive measure. Counterbalance is a time tested practice which can yield great health benefits.

Addressing Modern Day Issues

We live in a fast-paced world, facing constant pressures and great demands to produce within tight deadlines. Often there is little time to cook a proper meal. We eat on-the-go. We consume a diet of fast, processed food that is making many of us overweight. Our diets are too rich, containing excessive fat, sugar and carbohydrates. For many of us our diet is out of balance. We eat fattening foods with no opportunity to burn off the extra calories. We have a tendency to emphasize food taste and seldom consider whether it is healthy or not. Taste is further corrupted by the use of excessive salt, sugars and artificial flavorings.

For many, something is seriously wrong. Our affluent society's diet and lifestyle has made many of us less healthy than people living in much poorer countries. We all know about the usual reasons people attribute to good health: proper diet, exercise, relaxation and sleep. In spite of modern medicine, we as a whole are not as healthy as we should be. Most North Americans are overweight, many suffer from high anxiety and stress related problems and many suffer from chronic health problems, with prescription drugs the norm. What can we learn from the ancient Chinese culture that will enable us to live longer and healthier lives? What mistakes are we making that we are not even aware of and what can be done?

+ We are not eating foods that contain the proper nutrients that our bodies need.

+ The food that we eat often lacks the powerful plant based nutrients required to heal our bodies and to prevent many diseases. For example, scurvy was a major deficiency disease common among sailors, until it was discovered that vitamin C in citrus fruits like limes and oranges prevents and cures scurvy. Similarly there are other major deficiencies in our diets. This book gives a list of recipes and ingredients that traditional Chinese use to control such deficiencies.

+ We are not using our most powerful healing tool effectively, our own body.

+ The body has a natural ability to heal itself. The traditional Chinese way is to let the body heal itself first. Only if that fails, then medicine is prescribed. We must maintain a diet that is consistent with what our bodies need to heal and regenerate. We are what we eat. Know what is good for you and what is not. Pay attention to what you eat. Always consider what impact food is having upon your health.

+ We are eating the wrong food combinations. Our diets may include processed food and artificial ingredients to enhance taste. This type of food is hard for our systems to digest and may even slow metabolism. We do not know how to cleanse our bodily systems. A balanced diet entails combining something to cleanse and get rid of toxins and pollutants. As a result we should consider adding the following items to our diets: (unsweetened tea, more fruit, more green vegetables, legumes like taro, tofu and beans and health soups). Changing the food combinations can result in the desired changes.

+ Our diets are out of balance throwing our bodies out of balance. We have an undue emphasis on oily, greasy and sweet food. This emphasis is only on taste and not on health. We let our tongues overrule. Consider replacing these foods with fresh food that brings out the fresh natural taste cooked with little or no oil. Our diets are overly Yang (hot or *yit hay*), causing hot imbalances to develop within our bodies. Hot imbalances such as excessive acid can lead to chronic illnesses, by weakening the Yin (cooling or *leung*) that is responsible for healing and curing the body. Traditional Chinese Medicine states that aging is associated with the decline of the Yin function. Protecting the Yin shield is a major theme of both Chinese cooking and medicine. The Chinese culture emphasizes plant based food to help the body regulate itself.

• Our fast paced and stressful lives are causing us to age early and to die younger. We use vitamin pills to fight what ails us and even have special formulations for those over 50. While some believe that taking vitamin pills is ineffective because the body is unable to digest and absorb them, others believe that directly providing the body with these active ingredients will, over time, lessen the body's ability to produce special ingredients, thereby weakening the body's natural abilities. Traditional Chinese believe that the best way to obtain necessary vitamins is from the food we eat.

When one is overworked and overstressed, the Yang will overheat, eventually depleting the Yin and jing/essence [4].

One way to combat this problem is to make changes to our lifestyles to slow the pace to where we are comfortable and better able to manage our stress levels. The other way is to counterbalance the excessive Yang created by overwork and overstress with healing food.

Traditional Chinese believe that premature aging and early death is related to the depletion of the Yin and demise of the jing/essence. This is a key difference between our cultures. The Chinese are strong believers in the protective qualities of the Yin jing/essence. Western culture emphasizes the (Yang) external physical strength and places little emphasis upon the (Yin) internal healing aspects. The Chinese believe in providing the body with jing/essence from health soups and natural foods to prevent the demise of the jing/essence. The traditional Chinese strategy is to supply Yin or cooling essence to maintain the critical material needed for healing and rebuilding. In traditional Chinese medicine, health is equated with moisture and illness is equated with dryness. For example, people who are under stress may develop a dry cough. Certain moisturizing soups and drinks will alleviate this.

• We consume excessive amounts of unhealthy foods. There is a direct correlation between good health and proper diet. Yet we eat excessive amounts of food that does not promote health. Occasionally I come across people who love one type of food which throws their bodies out of balance and they do not even realize it. Some of the most common problems stem from: excessively Yang (hot or *yit hay*) food; greasy fat foods; excessively hot or spicy foods; food that does not agree with our bodily systems, and "junk foods".

Applying Traditional Chinese Practice

The type of food that we eat, combined with high pressure and fast moving lifestyles can often lead to health problems. In North America, more that one-half of its people are overweight or obese and suffer from various diseases like cancer, heart problems, diabetes and other problems at alarming levels. What is wrong with our diet and lifestyle? What can we learn from traditional Chinese diets and teachings to helping us to stay healthy and to live longer? There are major issues facing us:

We have improper diets. We are living in a place where food is abundant and relatively inexpensive. We tend to eat more than we need. For many the extra calories are translated into fat and obesity. It is important to eat fresh natural foods. The food we eat may contain artificial ingredients which are difficult to digest, slow metabolism and promote obesity. To improve our diets we need to consider the following:

+ Eat dark green vegetables every day.
+ Drink natural fruit and vegetable juices.
+ Learn how to prepare health soups that help the body regulate its internal balance, while providing essential healing jing/essences.
+ Eat more foods that heal and cleanse, such as tofu, watercress, winter melon, papayas.
+ Eat more natural food, such as fruit, vegetables, legumes.
+ Counterbalance fat, grease and excessive meat with dark tea which helps digestion and elimination.
+ Don't overeat.
+ Strive to be thin; slender people live longer.

We get insufficient exercise. For many of us, desk jobs and couch potato lifestyles are a serious problem. Many of us lack sufficient physical exercise leading to poor health. To improve our bodies we need to institute and maintain appropriate daily exercise programs.

Many of us are constantly overstressed. We are living in an era of high stress and high anxiety. We need to learn appropriate counterbalancing measures such as:

+ Getting sufficient sleep.
+ Developing self confidence and self control.
+ Exercising to relieve stress.
+ Being able to block out problems and allow the mind to relax.
+ Making care of health a top priority and realizing that health is the ultimate wealth.

We don't know how to eat properly. A most important part of traditional Chinese medicine is learning how to eat what is healthy. This entails:

+ Knowing what is good and what is not.
+ Making effective use of beneficial food.
+ Developing a taste for fresh natural ingredients and avoiding artificial products.
+ Eating moderately. Stop eating when you are still slightly hungry- don't overeat.
+ Eating a balanced diet to achieve and maintain a Yin Yang balance.
+ Drinking healthy beverages and health soups.
+ Eating foods that heal.

The traditional Chinese believe that health and vitality are protected by jing/essences and a proper diet may strengthen this vital resource, as well as preventing many illnesses. Certain foods contain jing/essences which are thought to be help the body's jing/essence. Eating food which contains the right jing/essences is deemed essential to good health. Knowing how food interacts is considered very important. We live in an era of food abundance, yet many are starved of the nutrients that can keep them healthy. Everyday new diets come out to help people lose weight, most untested. Maintaining an appropriate Yin Yang balance by eating foods that moisturize and cleanse is a time tested guideline for an effective eating strategy.

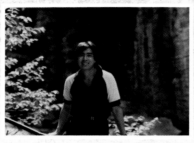

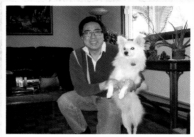

Joe Mah   1980   Joe Mah   2009

How Knowledge of the Universal Truth has Helped Me

The benefits of applying what I learned are obvious. People ask me how I don't seem to age. What do I know that they don't know? My knowledge of the Traditional Chinese teachings and dietary skills has served me well. After many years, it has become an inherent part of my life. I don't even think about it; I automatically counterbalance things. Yin Yang provides a valuable reference point for measurement. It sets the target of achieving harmony and balance as the way to good health.

I find that typical North American meals (such as steak, pork chops, mash, fries) are strong in the physical, external (Yang) aspects but weak in the healing, internal (Yin) aspects. I find applying the Yin (cooling or *leung*) aspects of my Chinese diet very useful in providing the jing/essences I need and that are missing from my North American diet. I have found that North American diets and Chinese diets may be combined to make a healthy fusion.

The traditional Chinese system implies discipline with moderation:

• Maintain a (Yin Yang) balance in both the body and the diet.
• Eat moderately.
• Provide adequate *yun* or moisturizing food to prevent dryness.
• Provide adequate *leung* (cool) jing/essences to minimize wear and tear.
• Eat food that helps cleanse and effectively remove toxins and wastes.

There are numerous imbalances and rebalancing is going on at all times within our bodies. This is normal. By being able to regulate the body's internal balance effectively, we have better control over our health.

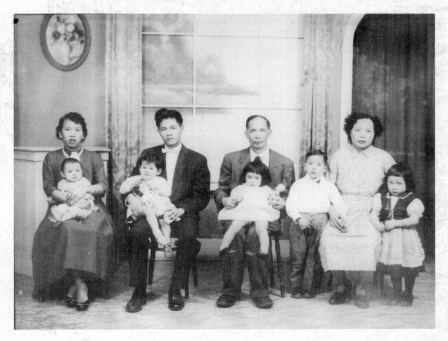

Mah Family 1957

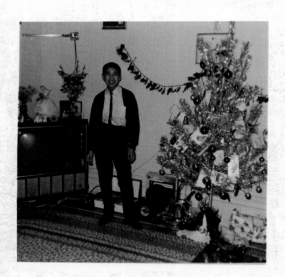

Joe Mah 1966

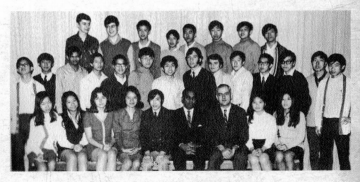

Montreal High School Chinese Club 1970
Joe Mah (president) - 1st row, 5th from the left

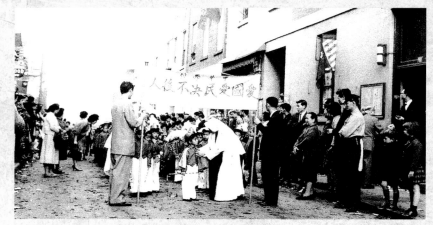

Chinatown Parade 1960's

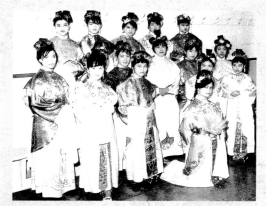

Chinese Dance Class 1965

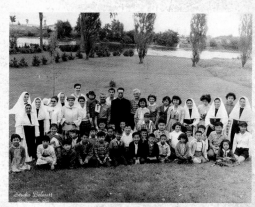

Chinese Summer School 1960's

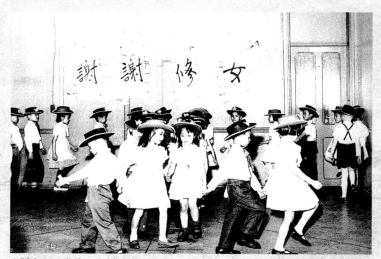

Chinese School 1960's

Growing up in Montreal's Chinatown in the 1950's and 60's

Chapter 2

Growing up in Montreal's Chinatown in the 1950's and 60's

Chinatown

This book resulted from training that I initially received at a very young age from a diverse group of people in Montreal's Chinatown during the 1950's and 60's. This training has been supplemented throughout my adult life, by practicing what I learned in childhood as an apprentice and continuing to consult with those who practise traditional Chinese medicine. Important lessons were learned from my parents, from Chinese herbalists with whom I apprenticed and from the real life experiences of growing up in a Canadian immigrant community. My training in traditional Chinese medicine, cooking and street smarts depends largely on the fact that I grew up in a community of first generation immigrants. These people grew up in the 1800's and were versed in traditional Chinese culture which had remained unchanged for thousands of years. These immigrants clung to the traditions of their homeland, preserving cultural concepts that often may even have been forgotten in the homeland. As a result, living in Montreal's Chinatown during my formative years provided me with an ideal setting for learning about traditional Chinese medicine and its reliance on appropriate food, dietary concepts and health soups.

I grew up in Montreal's Chinatown when it was a vibrant immigrant community. Cultural and social activities were centered around the Chinese associations- Wong Won Sun, Lee See, Hum Association, Chinese Benevolent Association and the local Chinese churches. Places of special importance to the recent immigrants were the Chinese herbalist stores- Wing Tai Chang, George Young's and Kuo Sing that provided remedies and consultations in traditional Chinese medicine. As well, grocery stores- Leong Jung, Sun Gon Worr, Foo Lon and Sun Sing

Lon provided many of the related ingredients. The local restaurants including the Nanking, New Lotus, Jade Garden, Sunya, Sun Kou Ming, Cathay, Ho Ho Café and Rickshaw Café were important meeting places.

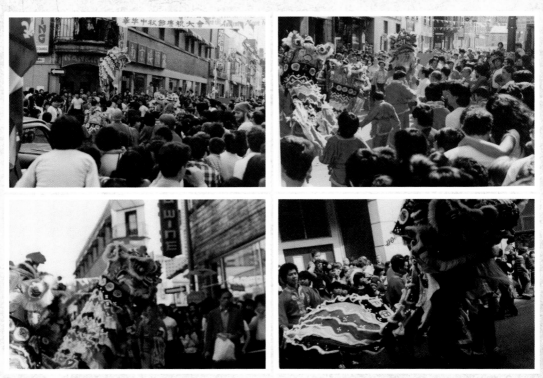

Montreal Chinatown October Lion Dance

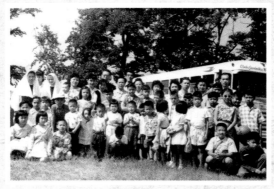

Chinese School Picnic 1962

Joe is third from left, front row

Memories from an Early Age

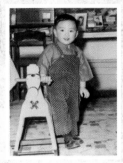

Joe Mah 1955

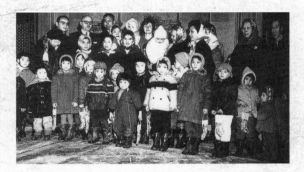

Chinese Catholic Mission Meeting with Rev. Thomas Tou and Montreal Mayor Jean Drapeau, City Hall, 1962. Joe Mah is first front left, followed his brother and two sisters.

source:
50th Anniversary of Rev. Tou's Appointment Booklet

I was born in Montreal's Chinatown in 1952. As a young child, I lived next door to a large, prominent Chinese cultural and political organization, with many aging members. I remember watching numerous funerals, for the average age of the membership was quite elderly, which made me keenly aware of how short life can be. Interestingly enough, I also remember that there were a number of elderly Chinese who were in extremely good health.

One day when I was about four years old as my father returned home from work he said that among the Chinese people there were those who knew the secrets of longevity. He said that he wanted me to learn these secrets as one of my missions in life. He noted that if I were successful in learning these secrets, I would be able to achieve everything that I wished and needed. As I grew I saw his logic that this was the right way. I bonded closely with my father as I watched him skillfully prepare meals, teaching me how to cook at a very early age.

My Parents

My parents both were excellent cooks who taught me how to make most of the health soups presented in this book and what the purpose was of each. They always prepared well-balanced meals and always included something to counteract any fat or grease in the meal. Maintaining an appropriate dietary balance by combining one type of food with another was an important daily exercise. My father always varied the meals, to provide both balance and variety. My initial training in *leung-yit* (cool-hot, Yin Yang) and herbal cures, as well as my cooking skills, came from my parents. My father also went to great lengths to introduce me at a young age to the small group of specialists in traditional Chinese medicine who practiced in Montreal's Chinatown. My father insisted that any training that I could receive in traditional Chinese medicine would be of great importance in my life as it would complement and build upon what I had learned at home.

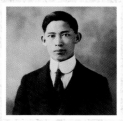

Dick Mah 1920's

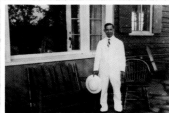

Dick Mah worked on a commercial farm during the 1930's

My father, Dick Mah, was born in China in 1895, in a village near Hong Kong and came to Canada in 1911 at the age of 16. In the following years he worked as a hired hand on a Quebec farm becoming very adept at growing Chinese vegetables. He started as a cook in Canadian railroad construction camps and later became a chef in North American and Chinese cuisine. My father became a well respected man in Montreal's Chinatown, largely because of the assistance that he provided to many during the Great Depression. At the time he was employed full time and was able to provide fresh vegetables and other assistance to many of the destitute unemployed.

My father was respected throughout the Chinese community and was able to call upon the local specialists in traditional Chinese medicine to teach me. I was fortunate in two respects: I had access to training from these specialists at an early age and I also had access to my father's background as an excellent chef.

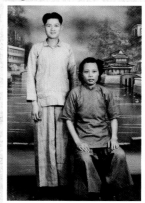

My mother Chew Chen Mah was also born in a village near Hong Kong in 1913 and came to Montreal's Chinatown in 1951. My parents were married in 1931 and I was born in 1952 into a family of two boys and two girls. We lived on Clark Street in Montreal's Chinatown.

Chew Chen Mah and cousin in 1950's

Lessons at Home

My father taught me cooking at a young age. My mother was also an excellent cook of traditional *Hoi San* cooking from Guangdong (Canton), China. They taught me the traditional Chinese concept of Yin Yang (*leung-yit*) meaning cooling-warming effects of food preparation and how an appropriate balance in the food we eat can impact health from childhood onward. *Leung-yit* is very prevalent in Chinese culture. I was told that this concept of maintaining Yin Yang balance had been a part of Chinese teachings for thousands of years.

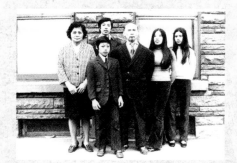

Family Picture in 1970

My parents stressed that certain wise people knew how to achieve good health and longevity and I should learn these secrets. They encouraged me to make understanding of these secrets a mission in life and that passing on this valuable knowledge to others should be a goal. They arranged for my training and apprenticeship with a number of Chinese experts and specialists, including practitioners in traditional Chinese medicine, herbal experts, health soup specialists, scholars and an elderly philosopher. These mentors taught me about Chinese cooking, culture, and philosophy. All of this would serve to complement my goal of learning how to live a longer and healthier life while slowing the aging process.

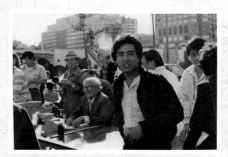

Joe Mah at Chinatown Festival 1978

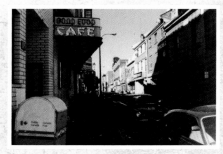

Montreal Chinatown 1970's

Lessons from Chinatown

I apprenticed (and "hung out" in my spare time) in several Chinese herbal stores. This was the traditional way of learning. These herbal stores were typical after-hours meeting places for those interested in all aspects of traditional Chinese medicine. I listened carefully whenever these specialists talked about Chinese health soups and their healing qualities. Even the Kung Fu experts (who also hung out) noted that Kung Fu is not a martial art as much as it is a regimen for maintaining bodily health. They observed that safeguarding health is of prime importance and stressed that cultivating internal peace and tranquility was tantamount and all were reluctant to use violence. They refused to teach potentially violent people or people with bad tempers. They trained me to be calm in the face of danger, to use logic, to respect the feelings of others and to allow people to save face to defuse conflicts. They emphasized the use of will power, mental strength and endurance in the face of trouble. They trained me to think

Growing up in Montreal's Chinatown in the 1950's and 60's

and act quickly. Valuable lessons are often learned by paying attention, being alert and being able to judge what is important and what is not. A valuable lesson could arise anytime, and most learn through listening and observing.

I was taught to control my temper and to remain cool and composed at all times, since one of the keys to good health and longevity is emotional control. Besides the obvious prevention of physical injuries, emotional outbreaks may create imbalances that injure the Qi (the life force) and also upset mental stability. The ability to control anger, fear, sadness, worry and even excessive happiness is important in maintaining a Yin Yang balance. In short, stay centered.

A wise person is able use the mind to balance life and to maintain stability. So it is not uncommon for the Chinese to reflect upon the bad times in the face of good times and to think of good times in the face of adversity. By maintaining stability you are always in control of the current situation. My mother often told me, that those who do not let anything bother them are able to live long healthy lives. Such people accept what life offers and are willing to live life regardless of its outcome. Under trying conditions, to be able to objectively analyze the situation at hand and to be able to act quickly and decisively without wasting time and energy on emotions is critical.

Today, people often ask me how I am able to stay looking so young and maintain such excellent health. Although I attribute part of this to my genetic makeup, the principal reason is living according to the teachings that I learned as a young apprentice in Chinatown and which I practiced and perfected during my adult life.

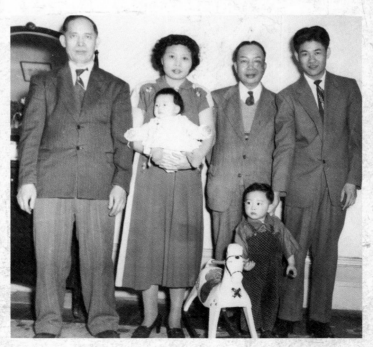

Mah Family and Relatives 1955

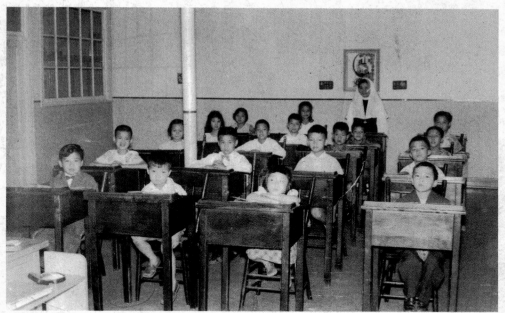

Chinese Class 1960, Joe Mah is seated
front right

Picture taken by Rev. Thomas Tou,   Montreal
Catholic Mission

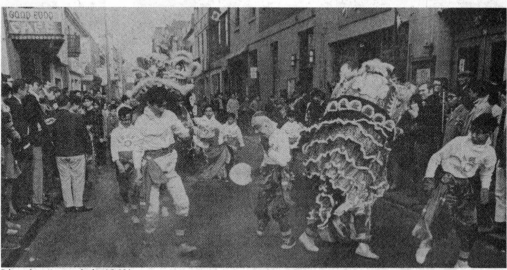

Lion dance parade in 1960's,
Joe Mah is the Teaser with mask

Source: Montreal Gazette Newspaper Clipping

Growing up in Montreal's Chinatown in the 1950's and 60's

An Introduction to George Young

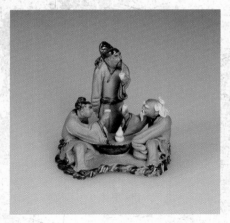

My parents asked George "Young Guy Buck" Young, an elderly Chinatown herbalist, to tutor me at age four. George was called the wise old man or *Lo Choon Bhu* of Chinatown. George taught me traditional Chinese culture such as the philosophies of *Tao Ti Ching* how to analyze and live life in a practical and effective manner. He had the corner store which sold soft drinks, cigarettes and Chinese herbal medicine. George was a herbal specialist and philosopher whom many Chinese came to consult. He had six chairs in his little store and every Sunday afternoon they would be filled with people taking part in discussions on a wide range of issues. I would arrive early every Sunday afternoon and would be given a choice of a little packaged cake or chips that he sold in his store. If I could sit patiently listening until late afternoon, I would be given a bottle of orange drink. There were no such drinks at home and I always stayed for my drink and usually longer because I became interested in the discussions, which dealt with Chinese culture, current events, health issues and philosophy. George Young had a deep understanding of the history, philosophy and the concepts of Yin Yang and taught me that these teachings must be used only as references or guidelines and not as absolute truths. This provided me with an important practical background in applying traditional Chinese medicine to enhancing health and promoting longevity. George Young also provided me with visual proof that following his practical approach will keep the body young and virile. He did so, when at age 88 he moved in with a voluptuous 40-year-old blonde who had been the toast of many Chinatown parties.

My apprenticeship to herbalist, Der Wing in his herbal store began at age eight. Der Wing taught me how to analyze illnesses caused by bodily imbalance, to use foods and soups to cure or offset illnesses, in the traditional Cantonese style using *leung-yit* (Yin Yang) concepts. He also taught me the importance of every item in the herbal store. Needless to say, much of my training was the result of listening to the discussions that Der Wing had with the visitors to his store.

Herbal expert, Mrs. Yee Tuh taught me about the importance of moisturizing soups and other liquid nutrients. She criticized the *leung-yit* concepts, indicating that they were not the most important issues. She further noted that this was a major shortcoming of traditional Chinese medicine. While *leung-yit* concepts may be appropriate for curing a specific illness, they are not necessarily appropriate as preventative measures to control the onset of disease. From her experience, she taught me that appropriate moisturizing and the use of essential nutrients were critical elements in maintaining bodily health. Her approach was to avoid a direct confrontation between *leung* (cold) and *yit* (hot), by using soups that are *worr* (neutral). She taught me that moisturizing neutral soups were key food components in maintaining bodily health. While herbal experts focus mainly on maintaining a *leung yit* balance, Mrs. Yee Tuh's teachings reinforced the body's constant need for *worr ping* (neutral peacefulness) regardless of the leung-yit condition.

The Three Wise Men

Sometime after meeting Der Wing, George Young and Mrs. Yee Tuh, my father asked if they had taught me the Chinese secrets of maintaining youth and longevity. Since I had not fully learned this valuable piece of Chinese knowledge; my father set out to find an expert in traditional Chinese medicine to teach me. Shortly thereafter, I was invited to sit outside on my street with three pleasant elderly Chinese. One of these men who looked rather distinguished, wearing a white suit and a hat was a Chinese herbal doctor. Another was Mr. Won Lee, a renowned scholar. The third was Mr. Wong a Chinese home medicine expert. They said that they would like to teach me the secrets of longevity if I would patiently sit and listen at their meetings.

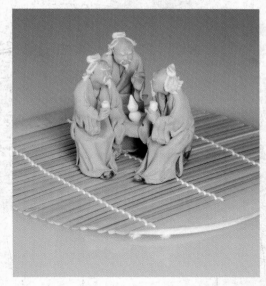

They began with a basic lesson on *leung-yit* and its impact on health. They stressed that *yit-hay* (excessive internal hotness) was a principal cause of illness and that such imbalances must be corrected quickly. The second most frequent cause of dietary illness was *ji* (bloating) from eating things that the body cannot *far-ji* (digest) and properly eliminate. When combined, these two problems cause major illness, as imbalance and blockage disrupt normal equilibrium. They taught me to remember this well and to pay close attention to the *leung-yit* balance. This was a different approach because most Chinese usually drink *leung* tea or soup when they become ill or when it is apparent that they have *yit-hay*. They taught me that management of the *leung-yit* balance was an ongoing process and not just an event that should be addressed when there is an apparent need. These men gave me valuable practical insights into a lifetime strategy to keep my body in balance to maintain good health and longevity. As time went on, I would sit and listen to them analyze various types of illnesses and their causes. I was very young and had never heard of these illnesses. They talked about how particular problems could have been avoided, about people who had died or were ill and what mistakes they had made in diet or in life style. Eventually, they told me that my lessons were complete and that I no longer had to sit with them, but that I was always welcome to join in, whenever I wished. So I continued to listen and to question. One of the most valuable lessons came from Mr. H. Won Lee, who taught me Yin Yang. His encouraging message and confidence inspired me, to achieve something in life.

Then one day the man with the white suit and hat no longer showed up and there were no more discussions about health and diet. I later learned that the man in white was a trained practitioner of traditional Chinese medicine and that he had opened a clinic for occidentals. Apparently a non-Chinese person who had become ill and who could not find a cure with Western medicine had come to see our friend. After an interview, it was concluded that the root cause of his illness was combined *yit-hay* (excessive internal heat) and *ji* (bloating), caused by an improper diet. The problem was corrected with a bag of Chinese *leung* herbal medicinal tea. This was the beginning of a busy occidental practice in traditional Chinese medicine for the man in the white suit.

The remaining two talked about how little Westerners know about *leung-yit*, and how they could live longer and healthier with its practice. In those days, the Chinese Canadians kept to themselves and they did not promote the Chinese culture outside of their community. Even amongst the Chinese themselves, the practitioners of traditional Chinese medicine were secretive. Training in its knowledge was valuable and these skills were not provided to just anyone. I was fortunate that my father had the appropriate connections in the Montreal Chinese community to enable me to receive this training.

In addition to my training from the man in the white suit and hat and his two partners, I received valuable assistance from a number of others, both as an apprentice and later in life, while I was practicing traditional Chinese home medicine. Mr. Yee, who was over 110 years old the last time we met, provided me with an assured proof of longevity if the tenets of *leung-yit* (cool-hot, Yin Yang) were followed. He also reinforced my reliance on drawing from the strength of nature itself. As well, Mr. Lee and several other Kung Fu masters revealed the importance of the three energies, the body's internal energy, associated with Yin; its physical energy, associated with Yang and its animate energy, associated with **Qi**.

Much later, my meetings with Thomas Hum served to reinforce my training in traditional Chinese medicine. Thomas is over eighty years old and still works six days a week at his food distribution business. Thomas has been studying Chinese healthcare since his teens. He confirmed that *worr-ping* or a neutral balance of the body to achieve a peaceful even state of mind and body is the overall objective. He said that what I was taught about moisturizing is correct. Moisturizing is neither *leung* nor *yit* (Yin nor Yang) but is neutral, and as such is important in balancing *leung yit* (cool-hot, Yin Yang).

Thomas said the Cantonese system of using food as medicine and a lifestyle of moderation are important preventive measures. Thomas said that Chinese healthcare practices are better at preventive medicine than Western. He said, if you can prevent illness and premature aging then medicine is not needed, regardless how old you are. However, if you are seriously ill, Western medicine is generally better because it goes after the problem directly. Operations to physically fix problems are much quicker and more effective than trying to induce the body to heal itself. The array of tools available to modern doctors and modern medical procedures are far more effective in treating an illness that has already taken root, than traditional Chinese medicine.

Benefits of My Apprenticeship

My knowledge of Chinese health concepts and soups has served me well over the years. People are often shocked when I tell them my age. Over the years, people often comment on how well I have preserved my health and reduced aging, asking me what is my secret. I credit a large part of my health, my slimness and my slow aging to the prudent use of the Chinese health soups discussed in the following chapters. Most people who experience internal health problems are missing the cool and moisturizing liquid nutrients essential to their internal organs and to healing and rebuilding their bodies. The Chinese have used soup as the main method of preventive healthcare for thousands of years. Health soup recipes were considered treasures and were passed from generation to generation. A family's knowledge of health soups was considered an intangible treasure and important when selecting a mate.

I recall hearing numerous discussions among Chinese people about how they improved their health or eliminated health problems by drinking certain soups. Soups were often the topics of discussion amongst my mother's friends. We exchanged soup recipes and stories with our Chinese friends as our soup making skills improved. As a young child returning home from school in the long cold winter, I looked forward to a bowl of old fashioned home style Chinese soup. My mother and her circle of friends all emphasized the importance of using extra ingredients to regulate and improve the health. Each soup had its unique health benefits. Soup ingredients were selected to help correct imbalance to prevent illness. The long boiled soups, which are presented in Chapters 6 to 8 are slow cooked- up to eight hours, using techniques similar to preparing herbal medications. I learned from a number of healthy elderly persons that these soups are essential to good health and longevity. As a result, I came to realize that soups can be successfully used as medicines and that health soups form an important part of traditional Chinese medicine.

One of my mother's friends Toy Ling Mah, who regularly visited us, passed away in December 2008, at the age of 105. She presents yet another example of how to live a long and healthy life. She drank Chinese soups, ate plenty of green vegetables, stayed active and maintained a focused outlook on life. While still in her eighties she readily accepted baby sitting assignments from her friends. Toy Ling Mah once told me to be happy and to always have something to live for. She added, "Look at your children's smiles; money cannot smile back at you. Look at all the good things in life and the achievements of this wonderful world." She concluded, "In life there will be times when the going gets tough; be strong and hang tough. Don't let circumstances get the better of you. Don't worry about problems. Instead do something about them. Have will power and determination. Visualize your success and achievements; work hard and there will be better days."

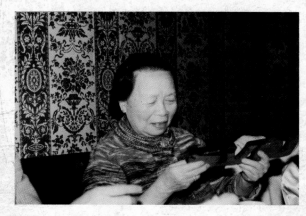

Toy Ling Mah lived to 105 years

Growing up in Montreal's Chinatown in the 1950's and 60's

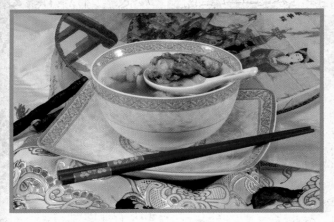

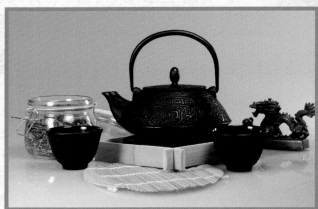

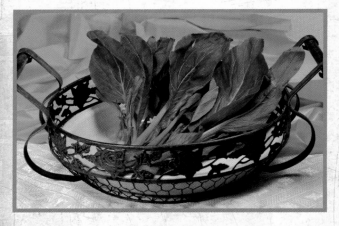

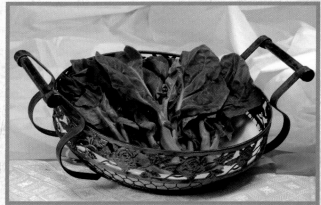

Introduction to Soup, Tea and Vegetables

Chapter 3

Introduction to Soup, Tea and Vegetables

A country's culture and philosophy are often best reflected through its cuisine. Understanding its food and diet provides an intimate view of Chinese culture, philosophy and the uniquely Chinese approach to health and life. In the first half of this book, ancient Chinese ideas and concepts are presented. But these thoughts are of limited value, unless you also know how to implement them. Implementation is contained in the second half of this book.

I have often been asked why some Asian people frequently appear young for their age. As well, I have been told that occidentals believe that Asians know special concepts about healthy living that are not taught in Western culture. I hope that this book will shed some light on these issues. As well, I have been told by a number of occidentals, that they are fascinated by the variety of foods offered in Chinese and Asian markets, and that they would dearly love to know what they are, how they are used and how to cook them. The objective of this book is to provide a practical understanding of Chinese health care practices and an answer some of the questions.

The Chinese have long used teas, special soups and vegetables to provide the essential nutrients needed to achieve *leung yit* (Yin Yang) balance, to cleanse the body of toxins, to slow aging, to prevent many diseases while helping the body heal and to manage weight. The second part of this book provides many recipes that have traditionally been used to promote balance and bodily health. This part of the book includes sections on teas, congees, quick boiled soups, long boiled soups, tonic soups, Ching Bo Leung health soups and Chinese vegetables.

Overview

Teas contain high concentrations of catechins, powerful antioxidants which are thought to be beneficial in disease prevention. Green tea contains chlorophyll, a renowned detoxifying agent with various vitamins. Teas are used to cleanse the body. They aid by neutralizing and eliminating greasy food residues.

Congees are great for breakfast, lunch or as a light snack. During cold days, a bowl of hot tasty congee warms the body and soothes the soul. Congees are often served during illness. Congees are low in calories and are used for weight control. Historically, congees were used during famines as the liquid fills the stomach, reducing hunger. Rice and other ingredients provide nutrients while the high liquid content helps to moisturize and cleanse the body.

Quick boiled soups are typically based on green vegetables. They contain high concentrations of dietary fiber that is essential in cleansing and elimination of waste. They contain chlorophyll, a renowned detoxification agent and the most basic food element found in nature.

Long boiled soups (*low for tong*) are prepared to extract powerful nutrients from the basic ingredients into the broth. When the hot liquid soup is ingested, it enters the blood stream with minimal need for digestion. Chinese herbalists believe that long boiled soups are the most effective way to deliver natural food nutrients. These soups contain many jing/essences, vitamins, minerals and natural sugars that help the body cleanse, heal and regain internal Yin Yang balance.

Tonic soups are specialty health soups which have been developed for special health objectives such as internal energy warming, internal energy cooling or addressing specific bodily needs.

Ching Bo Leung health soups are made from a combination of various natural food ingredients such as beans, seeds, fruits, nuts, vegetables and legumes. They are used to cleanse, detoxify and to regain *leung yit* (Yin Yang) balance. The Chinese have long used these soups for preventing illness. These soothing soups are often used during illness, to provide essential nutrients. These are the Chinese equivalents of chicken soup, and may be prepared with chicken stock.

Chinese green vegetables are available in Chinese and Asian markets. There is a large variety of green vegetables to choose from. They contain high concentrations of dietary fiber that is essential in cleansing and waste elimination. They also contain chlorophyll, a renowned detoxification agent. Traditional Chinese medicine teaches that a diet containing a large amount of dark green vegetables is essential for good health and longevity. Green vegetables are the key element in the *Ching Ting* (clear and natural) diet.

Ching Ting Diet

The *Ching Ting* (naturally clear and cleansing) diet is widely practiced by Chinese concerned about their health. Many healthy, elderly Chinese have adopted a practice of eating clear, natural food and maintaining weight. This diet provides broad guidelines on what and how much to eat. Only relatively low quantities of meat are consumed, whereas the diet has an excess of fresh green vegetables, which contain enzymes and dietary fiber that promote digestion and elimination. Those on this diet tend to be more selective with the food they eat, avoiding foods that are hard to digest as well as those that are overly greasy, hot or spicy. This type of diet contains powerful plant based nutrients called phytochemicals which heal and promote good health, as well as antioxidants for disease prevention.

The emphasis on plain, clear, naturally sweet food precludes the use of sweeteners or artificial flavorings. Generally very little oil is used in food preparation. Cool cooking methods such as steaming, boiling, poaching and light stir fried are used extensively. Hot or *yit hay* cooking methods, such as deep frying are seldom used. Many soup and vegetable recipes used in the *Ching Ting* diet are presented in this book. As the body ages, the metabolism and the digestive system slows down. The rate of metabolism may be increased and digestion improved through the consumption of fruits, vegetables and legumes while drinking plenty of juices, teas and soups.

Using Soups to Balance the Diet

The Chinese have long used soups as an important part of their diets and to maintain bodily balance. This practice of using health soups can potentially add years to your life and help avoid many illnesses. There are several possible solutions to each health issue and the answer is often a matter of trial and error. Each of us is different; what may work for one person may not necessarily work for another person. The Chinese believe that certain people have more hot (Yang) energy than cool (Yin) energy, which influences the degree of *leung yit* (Yin Yang) imbalance that can be tolerated. Conditioning and the previous use of certain foods also affect what a person can sustain. For example, people whose diets are normally hot and spicy are better able to deal with hot (Yang) energy excesses. East Indians who may eat excesses of hot curry (acidic) typically maintain a bodily balance by neutralizing the effects by consuming soothing yogurt (alkaline).

The Chinese road to good health is based upon balance and harmony. This requires eating a balanced diet that aids the body to help itself in quickly correcting imbalances. Knowing how to maintain bodily balance is key to living a long and healthy life. Considerable effort has been taken to present this valuable and complex subject in an easy to understand format to the reader.

Why do some Asians appear to age more slowly? Part of the answer is in the healing food and soups in their diets that protect the body. Knowledge of health soups is invaluable to safeguarding the body. The second part of this book presents many health soup recipes and a discussion of what they are generally thought to be good for. The Chinese believe that drinking an assortment of these soups can have good long term health benefits.

Yin Yang and Metabolism

Chinese herbalists believe that *yit hay* (hot imbalance) slows the body's metabolism and elimination. *Yit hay* (hot imbalance) is thought to cause indigestion, bloating, and constipation. *Leung* (cooling) food is thought to speed up metabolism, digestion and waste elimination.

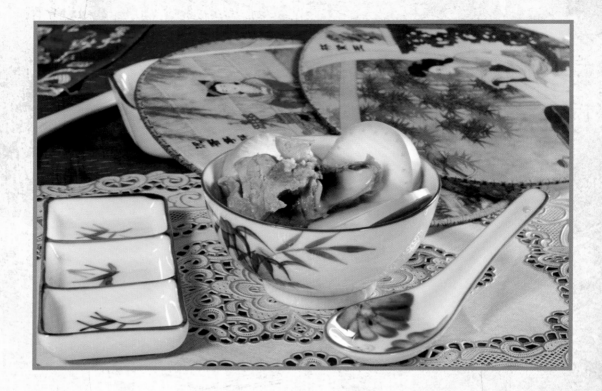

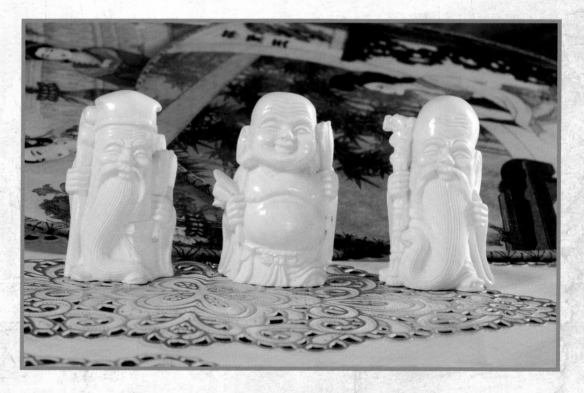

The Healing Properties of Chinese Health Soups

Chapter 4

The Healing Properties of Chinese Health Soups

The Role of Health Soups in Traditional Chinese Medicine

The Chinese have long used soups to heal the body. Over 5,000 years ago, the ancient Chinese classified the medicinal properties of hundreds of herbs and plants and began to prepare herbal tonics in soups that healed and nourished the human body. Essential nutrients and active ingredients were extracted from the herbs and food products by simply boiling them for extended periods. Over time, these preparations became part of the normal diet for most people. The resulting everyday health soups, until recently, were passed from generation to generation and their effectiveness was proven through this long and continued use. Unfortunately, in the modern age of fast foods and technological development, these teachings of traditional Chinese medicine are being forgotten or overlooked, both in China and in the Western world. Even amongst the Chinese, most do not know exactly what each soup is good for.

Traditional Chinese medicine considers soups as the best medium for delivering both nutrition and healing essences to the human body because they provide natural nutrients which are easily absorbed and which can quickly be used by the body to heal itself. Soups nourish and cleanse the body, promoting digestion and elimination. Certain soups moisturize the body by triggering its internal systems to stay moist. Soups can provide critical moisturizing essences together with highly concentrated nutrients in an easily utilized form. Ancient Chinese teachings support modern medical understanding which recognizes that the human body uses fluids to deliver nutrition to the cells and to remove their waste. In liquid form, nutrients and other active ingredients are delivered into the bloodstream quickly and efficiently, whereas when supplied in solid food, digestion must first take place.

Two basic types of Chinese health soups are presented; traditional long boiled (*low for tong*) soups and the quick boiled soups. The traditional long boiled health soups are prepared using special lengthened cooking procedures that extract the maximum nutritive value from the base ingredients into the soup stock, while the quick boiled soups use a much shorter preparation time. Normally only the liquid stock from long boiled soups is consumed and any remaining solids are discarded, since most of the nutritive value is removed from the solids in the long boiling process. All of the ingredients of quick boiled soups are consumed. Simple Chinese health soups not only soothe the body, they ease internal irritation. Soups prevent constipation while speeding digestion and elimination, because they fill the stomach with the fluids that it needs to digest other solid food. A diet consisting of a high concentration of healthy soups is also a simple, effective way of controlling and maintaining a suitable body weight, since the body does not feel hungry when the stomach is filled with fluids.

Using soups to prevent and cure illness is a basic tenet of traditional Chinese medicine. Maintaining good health through an appropriate diet eliminates the need for strong medicines with their possible side effects. Provided that there are no allergic reactions to any of their components, health soups have no side effects.

Soups and their uses were a most important part of traditional Chinese medicine because they provided the basic methods of staying healthy and overcoming illnesses. The preparation of long boiled soups almost became an art form. Recipes were passed down from generation to generation. It used to be considered a sign of love and affection to prepare a good healthy soup for the family and its friends. It took skill, practice, time and effort to make healthy and tasty soups. As was discussed above, much of this important background is quickly being forgotten or ignored in this age of fast foods. It is hoped this book will help preserve an important part of this history for future generations.

Soups with Cooling and Moisturizing Essences

Soups with *leung* (cooling) essences and with *yun* (moisturizing) essences are served as a part of traditional Chinese home-style meals to help maintain bodily strength and health. Traditional Chinese, many of whom are found in immigrant communities around the world, believe that the body needs to consume such cooling and moisturizing essences on an ongoing basis and as a result they must be constantly replaced. The teachings of traditional Chinese medicine are that these valuable essences should be replaced by drinking appropriate health soups that have proven their effectiveness over many generations. If a diet lacks these cooling and moisturizing essences, the body is not equipped to properly repair and heal itself.

Traditional Chinese consider that drinking water alone is inadequate. Soups, teas and juices are considered to have better healing powers than water. However, the body also needs water to rebuild. Once you learn to appreciate the natural taste of health soups, you will actually notice and experience their soothing effects while you are drinking them. As shown below, there are many types of soups containing cooling and moisturizing essences; each type provides specific beneficial effects. Traditional Chinese often tailor their soups specifically to counteract possible negative attributes of the meal being served. For example, if a meal contains foods with excessive amounts of *yit* (warming) essences, such as deep fried or barbequed food, a soup with appropriate *leung* (cooling) essences is used to help maintain an appropriate *leung-yit* bodily balance. This technique prevents a possible bodily imbalance caused by excessive consumption of foods that contain only warming essences. The traditional Chinese refer to excessive *yit* or hot diet driven imbalance as *yit hay*.

Health soups with *leung* (cooling) and *yun* (moisturizing) essences help the body in several different ways. While promoting internal bodily balance as described above, they also assist in the breakdown of fats and grease, while promoting digestion and waste elimination. Certain health soups provide moisturizing nutrients that soothe and heal. Soups with cooling and moisturizing essences are often prescribed by traditional Chinese herbalists to prevent and cure illnesses that are caused by bodily imbalance. Five of the most popular and beneficial long boiled soups are: *ching bo leung*, winter melon with mung beans, cole, watercress, and carrots with black turtle beans. I drink these soups regularly.

Some Basic Soup Making Instructions and Facts

Although specific instructions for making a number of special health soups are presented below, there are some basic instructions that apply to all these soups.

All special soup ingredients are available at Chinese or Asian food stores or at Chinese herbal health food stores. Many other more common ingredients are available in conventional supermarkets. Some of the more popular health soups may even be available as a pre-mixed herbal package which is then combined with fresh vegetables and meats as required. It is important to read the ingredients on such pre-mixed packages to ensure that all the required ingredients are included.

Soups are an excellent dietary measure for weight control. Soups are mainly water and when the stomach is filled with such a liquid, its craving for other food is effectively controlled. For this reason, it is important that any remaining fat or grease be skimmed off the surface of all soups before serving. An easy method to remove all the fat from a soup is to first chill the soup and allow the grease to harden. It can then quickly be removed with a strainer. In traditional long boiled health soups, all the beneficial nutrients are transferred into the liquid stock from the base components; base ingredients and especially any meats (except seafood, ox-tail and abalone) are often discarded before drinking the soup. The caloric content of traditional long boiled soups is very low since only the soup stock is consumed.

The cooking times for long boiled soups are based upon bringing the soup to an initial boil and reducing the heat to allow the soup to simmer. Several options are then possible. The soup can be allowed to simmer for the specified time, where the soup is gently bubbling. However after initial boiling, the cooking temperature can lowered to 80 °C (175 °F) and the specified cooking time increased by 50%. A slow cooker may also be used to make these soups. Start with boiling water and then set the slow cooker for about 14 to 16 hours at low heat, or 10 to 12 hours at medium heat. This will vary, depending on the individual slow cooker.

Most of the listed soups normally have some meat as a base ingredient. Soups can become vegetarian by simply not adding any meat. All soups which have herbal ingredients normally require some meat, to take the edge off the herbal taste. Otherwise, the resulting stock may not be very palatable or tasty and could even cause irritation. Chinese herbalists believe that meat and bones provide Yin Yang balance to the soup by counterbalancing the herbal or vegetable ingredients.

This book presents recipes for a number of traditional long boiled soups and quick boiled soups. This is followed by two shorter sections which provide recipes for traditional congees and a description of traditional teas. Listed with each soup recipe, is a description of the types of essences provided by the soup, and its represented health benefits.

The Importance of Taste and Smell in Soup Preparation

The taste, smell and known freshness of all ingredients play an important role in cooking effective and tasty health soups. A good soup can always be identified by its natural taste and related aroma. Long-boiled health soups are allowed to simmer for hours to extract the natural ingredients into the soup stock. Only once the natural taste has been developed, are you certain that all the healing nutrients have been extracted from the base ingredients into the soup stock. If the natural taste and aroma have not been developed, nutrients are still locked within the base ingredients and the full health benefits are not yet available. Once the taste and aroma have fully developed such long boiled health soups are drunk like a tea, since the base ingredients become empty of nutrition and are discarded. The taste, smell and freshness of the base ingredients are the outward signs of their ability to provide healthy nutrients. For this reason, traditional, home-style Chinese cuisine does not include artificial food additives, taste enhancers like monosodium glutamate (MSG), strong spices or sweeteners. All such additives simply mask the natural taste of the base ingredients. To get great taste and maximum health benefits, it is important to start with good quality fresh food ingredients, especially with seafood, meat, bones and vegetables.

The taste will tell. By tasting a soup as it simmers, you can tell when it is ready to serve. The taste of a good soup is natural and reflects the nature of its base ingredients; it is not masked or distorted by artificial additives. A cook who uses artificial ingredients to enhance a soup is considered mediocre and as someone more concerned with taste than with health. The best health soups are usually the ones you make yourself. Once you learn how, it is so easy to make great tasting health soups. These are some of the most valuable skills you will ever learn to maintain and improve your bodily health. They also will help to promote longevity and well-being.

Appropriately Using Soups to Regulate Health

Health soups are not intended to be used as an alternative to modern medical healthcare. Traditional Chinese drink health soups for preventive health purposes, much like taking vitamins. Each soup presented provides a different set of nutrients. Each soup has its own unique health benefits. To obtain their optimum health benefits, these soups must be appropriately incorporated into your daily diet. You must learn to gage what is happening within your own body, to comprehend potential health issues and to select the appropriate soup to counterbalance a problem or simply to supply yourself with appropriate preventative nutrients.

Providing Internal Moisturizing

Soups with *yun* (moisturizing) essences prevent inner bodily dryness and related health problems. Moisturizing assists the body to heal itself and to rebuild. Moisturizing ingredients include: *luo han guo*, sugar cane, carrots, arrowroot and honey dates. Honey, fresh oranges and orange juice are also moisturizing. *Yun fay* (deep moisturizing of the lungs) helps the *Qi* (breathing) and improves health. Providing the body with adequate *yun fay* (deep moisturizing of the lungs) nutrients is important in helping you stay young. Internal dryness like external dryness causes premature aging. Internal dryness is thought to be the root cause of many illnesses.

Yin Yang and Health

The Chinese use Yin Yang in different ways for both health and exercise purposes. Both Kung Fu masters and traditional Chinese medicine experts take Yin Yang and *Qi* into consideration.

1. Principle Bodily Energies as Practiced in Kung Fu

In Kung Fu, internal energy (such as pulse) is related to Yin, physical energy is related to Yang and animate (breath) energy is related to *Qi*. As a result there are three basic types of Kung Fu:

- Hard or physical Kung Fu such as *Wing Chun* is related to Yang.
- *Tai Chi Chuan* which focuses on using soft or internal energy is related to Yin.
- *Chi Gong* which focuses on breathing is related to *Qi*.

2. Principle Bodily Energies in Chinese Medicine

Yin, Yang and *Qi* are associated with bodily energies in traditional Chinese medicine:

- Healing ability and body rebuilding are related to Yin.
- Physical energy and muscle power are related to Yang.
- Breathing or animate energy is related to *Qi*.

In North America, with its rich diet and good medical care, people tend to be physically strong, large and overweight. Their illnesses do not generally result from malnutrition. Their bodies are strong and can normally address external stress. Their tendency is to have illnesses related to their excessive size and weight; as well as lack of jing/essences that help heal the body. Their illnesses tend to be internal, such as high blood pressure and diabetes. In Chinese terms, they have excessive Yang energy and insufficient Yin energy to counterbalance it. Knowledge of Chinese methods to achieve balance can be useful.

In places where people eat a basic fruit, vegetable and whole grain diet with fewer animal products, people do not have problems associated with eating excessive fat, meat and processed foods. Their plant based diets provide them with plant based healing nutrients. On the other hand, in places with malnutrition and lack of medical care, people suffer from insufficient Yang energy and many of their illnesses tend to be physical or external in nature.

3. Internal Energy Balance

We typically measure vital signs such as heart rate, blood pressure and temperature to determine our bodily condition. The Chinese consider *leung-yit* (cold-hot, Yin Yang) balance as an additional key vital sign. *Leung-yit* characterizes the body's internal energy balance. In the Chinese culture, internal energy imbalance is a precursor to many bodily problems. Imbalance may be the result of *leung* (cooling, Yin) conditions or *yit hay* (hot or Yang) conditions. *Leung-yit* is deeply rooted in the Chinese culture but largely unknown elsewhere. It is all about balancing food properties with bodily condition.

Food and diet have a profound impact upon the body's condition and its *leung-yit* balance. For example, food affects the body's pH balance. *Yit hay* food combined with hot preparation methods (deep frying, barbequing) may cause excessive acidity within the body. By eating too much hot, spicy food, you may develop hot breath or *yit hay*. However, each of us is unique and must deal with *leung-yit* in a personal manner.

According to ancient Chinese wisdom, the key to good health is *leung-yit* balance. When the body is in equilibrium, it is positioned to heal and rebuild itself. Food and health soups are used to supplement the body with required jing/essence.

Periodic short term *leung-yit* imbalance is normal. The body automatically rebalances itself over time. But persistent long term *yit hay* is thought to cause premature aging and to be the root cause of many chronic illnesses. Knowledgeable Chinese take the *leung-yit* balance of their body seriously and adjust their daily diet accordingly. A proper meal is *leung-yit* balanced. *Leung* items are included in meals to offset *yit* food. For example, if you have *yit hay* imbalance, you should lower your intake or abstain from such foods. You should increase the amount of *leung* foods such as fruits, vegetables, legumes, green tea, juice and *leung* soups (there are many recipes in this book) to counterbalance the *yit*.

Cold or *Leung* Imbalance Symptoms

Cold or *leung* internal energy imbalance is associated with yin. It can be caused by:

+ **Yin Yang (*leung-yit*) Imbalances:** diet imbalance, excessive cold (*leung*) food and/or lack of warming (*yit*) food.

+ **Nutritional Factors:** poor nutrition, lack of meat and/or protein in the diet, lack of iron, poor eating habits and starvation.

+ **Internal Factors:** poor mental or physical health, high stress, mental distress, depression, old age and illness.

+ **External Factors:** a cold environment or cold weather.

In a cold (*leung*) imbalance, there is a lack of warm (*yit*) internal heat or fire. This condition is also known as *shill for* (shortage of internal heat or fire). Physical signs include chills, a pale complexion, bitter saliva and general weakness. Soups containing *yit* (warming) essences are used to offset such imbalances and to strengthen the body. Meat consumption may be increased to strengthen the body as well. This type of imbalance is far more serious than a *yit hay* or hot imbalance.

Hot or *Yit Hay* Imbalance Symptoms

The opposite of a cold (*leung*) imbalance is a hot (*yit hay*) internal heat imbalance. *Yit hay* which literally means hot breath is much more common. When there is an excess of hot internal energy or *yit hay*, the body may be overheated and dry. Causes of hot (*yit hay*) imbalance:

+ **Yin Yang (*leung-yit*) Imbalances:** diet imbalance, excessive hot (*yit hay*) food and/or lack of cooling (*leung*) food.

+ **Nutritional Factors:** consumption of excessive amounts of hot(*yit hay*) food and/or food cooked using hot cooking methods, such as deep frying, grilling and excessive alcohol consumption.

- ✦ **Internal Factors:** illness, hot temper, being emotionally upset and excitement.
- ✦ **External Factors:** a hot dry environment or hot weather.

Yit hay (hot imbalance) symptoms include: hot smelly breath, excessive thirst, red rash, dry mouth, dry skin, dark yellow urine and constipation. If there is phlegm (mucous), white is considered *leung* (cold) and yellow is considered *yit hay* (hot). Normally the body adjusts and eventually gets itself back into balance. This is normally not a serious problem, but to Chinese herbalists, chronic *yit hay* is the root of eventual chronic illnesses. The strategy is to take care of *yit hay* on a regular and ongoing basis, by reducing or eliminating its cause such as hot spicy food, deep fried food and to increase cooling food and to drink soups which help restore internal balance.

Soups with *yun* (moisturizing) and *leung* (cooling) essences are used to stimulate moisturizing and to restore bodily balance. Herbalists believe that when there is a major imbalance, the body's healing energies are used to restore balance and may hamper healing. Providing balance helps the body to heal. The long boiled soup recipes in this book are mostly neutral, and are good are regulating and restoring both *leung* (cold) and *yit hay* (hot) imbalances. They are best when used for preventive purposes rather than corrective purposes.

Finally, the body's animate energy and lung function can be assisted and enhanced with several different soups that strengthen breathing, clear the lungs and reduce phlegm (mucous) accumulation. This is known as maintaining a *qi* (*hay*) balance. Soups are used to help strengthen the *qi* (breathing), lower the *qi*, cleanse the *qi* and most importantly to moisturize the *qi* or *yun fay* (deep lubrication of the lungs). Reducing phlegm (mucous) and clearing chest congestion or "*far hum- do qi*" are important objectives of health soups and herbal teas.

Other Benefits of Health Soups

Benefits gained from the appropriate use of health soups include:
- ✦ Promoting digestion, elimination and bodily cleansing.
- ✦ Providing soothing, healing and balancing affects on the digestive system.
- ✦ Strengthening the kidney and bladder system.
- ✦ Adding calcium to the diet from the soup bones.
- ✦ Providing the building block materials needed to restore and heal tendons and joints from ingredients such as pig knuckles, ox-tail and fish bladders.
- ✦ Providing preventative health qualities, such as reducing cholesterol, controlling body weight and improving heart problems.
- ✦ Providing the body with powerful plant and herbal based healing essences.

Healing Properties of Some Typical Ingredients of Health Soups

Traditional Chinese health soups contain various special herbs and plant and animal materials which in combination produce special beneficial effects. These overall effects result from the unique properties of each ingredient.

Ching Bo Leung (Say Mee) Ingredients

The following ingredients are used in many Chinese soup recipes.

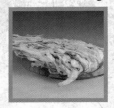

Polygonatum (Solomon's Seal)

Polygonatum provides *yun* (cooling) moisturizing essences.

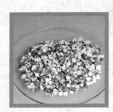

Fox Nuts (*Sze Sek*)

Fox nuts provide mild *leung* (cooling) essences and are thought to have healing qualities.

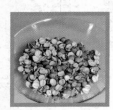

Lotus Seeds

Lotus seeds provide *leung* (cooling) essences and are thought to be good for the skin and the complexion.

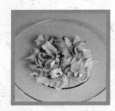

Dried Lily Bulbs

Dried lily bulbs provide *leung* (cooling) and moisturizing essences which aid in overcoming dryness and thirst.

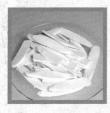

Dioscorea (Chinese Yam)

Dioscorea provides neutral, soothing essences that assist with internal bodily balance. It is thought to reinforce the *qi* (breathing) and is good for the kidneys. It is used to help relieve coughing and poor appetite.

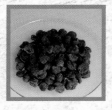

Dried Longan

Longan in Chinese means dragon eye. Dried longan provides both neutral and moisturizing essences. It promotes a good appetite and its soothing sweetness provides special plant sugars to assist in bodily rebuilding. It contains magnesium, phosphorus, vitamins A and C. It is thought to be good for the blood and heart.

Barley

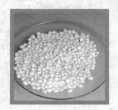

Hulled or pearled barley provides neutral essences that promote internal cleansing and bodily balance. It is especially soothing in relieving chills which may be precursors to a cold. It is good for the digestive system and the stomach. Popped barley (as shown) is also available.

Wolfberry Seeds (Goji, Gigi, Lycium barbarum)

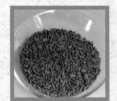

Chinese herbalists believe that these seeds have *Boo* or strengthening properties. They are thought to help healing and to provide good protective properties, especially for the eyes, when cooked with liver. Western culture is beginning to recognize this fruit as an important health food. It is available in many health food stores and is eaten as a sweet seed, like a dried berry. For Chinese herbalists, the best way to get these nutrients is in a soup. Wolfberries have been used in Chinese medicine for thousands of years. Wolfberries are orange in color and contain beta-carotene, lutein, and zeaxanthin which are generally thought to be good for the eyes. Chinese herbal shops usually carry larger and higher grade wolfberry seeds than those available at Asian supermarkets.

Luo Han Guo (Lo Hon Fruit, Siraitia grosvenorii)

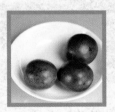

Luo Han Guo is very sweet, and is about 300 times sweeter than sugar by weight. It has been used by the Chinese as a natural sweetener for over 1,000 years. It is a member of the gourd family and has long been used as a longevity aid. The entire fruit is used and only a small amount, a tablespoon is used at a time. If a large amount is used, it darkens a soup and gives the soup a strong herbal medicine taste. Chinese herbalists have long used luo han guo for its preventive properties. Herbalist Mrs. Yee said this was one of the most effective healing sugars. It is *yun fay* (lubricates the lungs) which also helps healing and is used to help the body to stay young. It is often used in Chinese medicine for coughs and treatment of internal dryness.

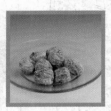

Dried Honey Dates

Honey dates are sweet and moisturizing, and help fight dryness. Their lubricating properties are thought to be beneficial to the face and skin.

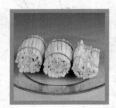

Sand Ginseng (Glehnia Root)

Sand ginseng comes in small thin sticks and larger sizes. It is bitter sweet tasting. It affects the stomach and lungs. It is *leung* (cooling) and *yun* (moisturizing).

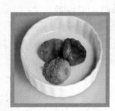

Dried Figs

Figs are very sweet and have moisturizing qualities.

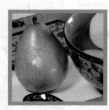

Pears

Pears are sweet and have moisturizing qualities. Pears are mildly *leung* (cooling) and help reduce *yit hay* or internal heat. They are good for coughs and indigestion. Pears help produce fluids that lubricate dryness. Pears have natural sugars which help cleansing, digestion and elimination.

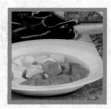

Carrots

Carrots may be added to Ching Bo Leung soup, giving it a sweet carrot taste. Carrots have many health benefits. Carrots in soup are soothing, especially when you have a cold or the flu. Carrots are renowned to be good for the eyes and contain vitamins A, B6 and C as well as magnesium, iron, calcium and niacin.

Apricot Pits

Apricot pits reduce phlegm (*far hum do hay*), ease breathing, and suppress coughing. There are two types: Northern and Southern. Northern (*buck hung*) apricot pits are bitter. They are *leung* (cooling) and are used for *yit hay* (hot imbalance) or when there is yellowish phlegm. Southern (*nam hung*) apricot pits are sweet. They are slightly *yit* (warming) and are used for *leung* (cold imbalance) or whitish phlegm.

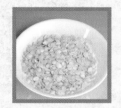

Regular almonds, available at all supermarkets, may be used as a substitute for apricot pits.

A 50-50 blend of Northern (*buck hung*, bitter) apricot pits and Southern (*nam hung*, sweet) apricot pits may also be used.

Warning:

Raw apricot pits are a mild poison. Do not use raw apricot seeds or pits. Buy cooked or processed apricot pits from reputable stores. Do not use excessive amounts of northern apricot pits; they are bitter and may be harmful in large quantities. If there are any safety concerns, use almonds, instead.

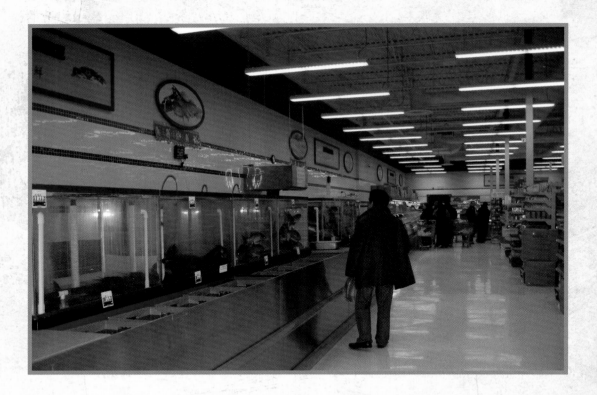

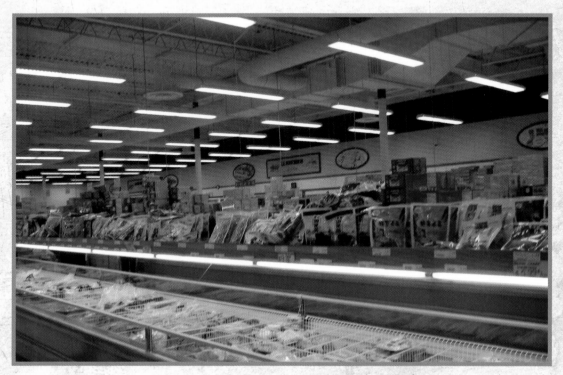

Kim Phat Market in Montreal, Canada

Chapter 5

A Trip to the Chinese/Asian Market

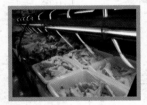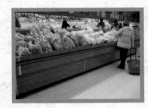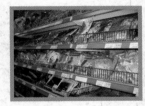

I n traditional Chinese medicine, there is direct correlation between food and health. Knowing the health properties of each ingredient, how to prepare the ingredient and when to use it is considered sacred knowledge. This knowledge has been passed from generation to generation and remains an important part of the practice of traditional Chinese medicine. Effective use of Chinese health soups depends upon the use of appropriate ingredients that can be readily obtained. This chapter discusses soup ingredients, their properties and health benefits and where to obtain them. As is seen, many components are available in typical North American supermarkets, while special ingredients are available from Chinese supermarkets that are a part of most North American cities.

Using Meat

Meats such as beef, pork, chicken or lamb are important ingredients in most Chinese health soups. Since all the solid ingredients, including any meat or bones, are discarded after the lengthy slow cooking process leaving only the broth, preparation of health soups can be relatively inexpensive. Soup bones, beef shanks, pig's knuckles, stew meat and brisket are normally used instead of expensive cuts of meat. Oxtail is also a traditional tasty meat that is used extensively in Chinese health soups. Meats add essential nutritive ingredients to long boiled soups and add protein to fast boiled soups.

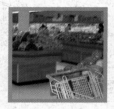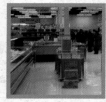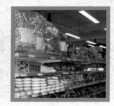

Using Bones and Cartilage

Chinese use soup bones extensively. Bones provide needed calcium, especially as you get older. So instead of taking calcium pills, the Chinese make soups with bones, such as pork bones or chicken bones. With the occurrence of mad cow disease, beef bones are used less frequently. When I buy oxtail, I select small tails from young cattle. The Chinese also use tendons such as found in oxtail and pig knuckles to strengthen tendons, joints, and cartilage, especially as you get older.

Using Offals

Some ingredients such as heart, liver and kidneys, which many people discard, are considered by the Chinese to be healthy delicacies. Heart is thought to strengthen the heart, while liver is considered to strengthen the liver and to treat eye problems. (The eyes and liver are thought to share a Yin Yang relationship. When you have jaundice (a liver problem) the eyes become yellow.) Kidneys are thought to strengthen the kidneys. The Chinese believe that the kidneys are the main storage of jing/essence and protecting the kidneys is a key preventive strategy.

All required meat ingredients are readily available in conventional butcher shops and supermarkets. They also are available in most North American Chinese markets.

Using Seafood and Seaweed

Scallops, oysters, clams, shrimp, squid, octopus and related common seafood items are often used in health soups. In fresh or frozen forms they are readily available from fish stores or supermarkets; while in dried, pre-packaged forms, they are available at Chinese markets. Seafood provides a combination of nourishing ingredients. Some special seafood items such as abalone, conch and seaweed are available in Chinese or Asian markets.

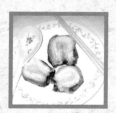

Abalone
Abalone, a shellfish, is available in dried, canned or frozen forms. Abalone is reported to help control urination and to strengthen the bladder. Abalone is not recommended for those with heart problems.

Conch

Fresh, frozen or dried conch normally is available at larger Asian markets. It is thought to be good for the kidneys and bladder; it is reported to help control urination and to strengthen the bladder.

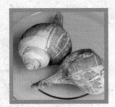

Seaweed (Laver)

Many types of dried seaweed are available as pre-packaged items. Seaweed is *leung* (cooling) and assists in cleansing the digestive system. Seaweed speeds digestion and elimination.

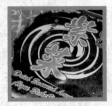

Black Fungus (*Fhat Choy* or hair vegetable)

Black fungus is a special type of seaweed that that resembles black hair. It is thought to aid digestion. It may sometimes be difficult to find in the market. The name *fhat choy* sounds like 'get rich' and is a popular item during New Year's celebrations.

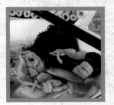

Using Beans and Tofu

The following is a short list of some bean and tofu items used in traditional health soups. All are normally available from North American Asian markets and many are available in traditional supermarkets.

Dried Bean Curd

Dried bean curd (dried tofu) is available in 170 g (6oz) packages in either sheet or stick form. The stick type is normally used for long boiled health soups. Bean curd is made from soya beans, is high in protein and has good preventive health properties. It is a highly recommended health food item.

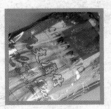

Fresh Bean Curd (Tofu)

Fresh tofu is locally made in most North American cities and is readily available. It is high in protein, has good preventive health properties and is a highly recommended health food item. It is also available in vacuum sealed packages that do not require refrigeration.

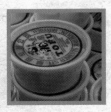

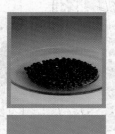

Black Turtle Beans

These beans are beneficial to the **Qi** (breath) and reputedly strengthen the body's breathing capacity. They also have high protein content. Black Turtle Beans are considered to have *leung* (cooling) properties. Some elderly Chinese panfry raw black turtle beans before using them in soup as this neutralizes the *leung* (cooling) aspects.

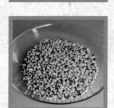

Black Eyed Peas

These beans are also beneficial to the **Qi** (breath) and reputedly strengthen the body's breathing capacity. They also have high protein content.

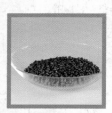

Red Mung Beans

These beans are beneficial in bodily healing. Red mung beans are a staple ingredient of Chinese food medicine and are regarded as having essential nutrients to aid the body in overcoming illness. They are considered to have slightly *yit* (hot or heating) properties. They are commonly used to combat *leung* (cold) illnesses and are high in protein.

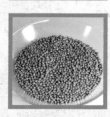

Green Mung Beans

These beans are beneficial in healing the body and in assisting the body to rid itself of accumulated *yit doak* (hot toxins). Green mung beans are a staple ingredient of Chinese food medicine and are regarded as having essential nutrients to aid the body in overcoming illness. Green mung beans are *leung* (cooling). They are commonly used in combating a *yit hay* (hot imbalance) illness and are high in protein. They are also used to overcome skin problems and rashes.

Using Fruit, Sweeteners and Flavorings

The following shows some fruit, fruit products, sweeteners and flavorings used in traditional health soups. All are normally available from Asian supermarkets.

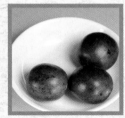

Dried Longan

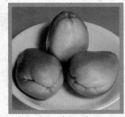

Luo Han Guo

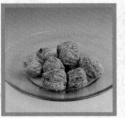

Dried Figs

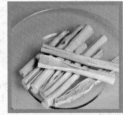

Chayote (Sechium edule)

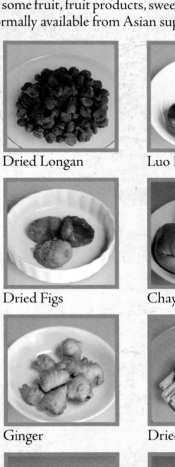

Ginger

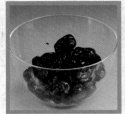

Dried Sugar Cane

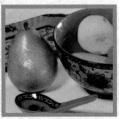

Chinese Honey Dates

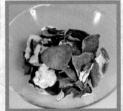

Chinese Red Dates
(Jujube)

Pear and Apple

Mandarin or Tangerine Peel

A Trip to the Chinese/Asian Market

Using Dried Seafood

Dried seafood such as dried shrimps, scallops, and fish maw are often used to make soup. The drying process gives the seafood a deep tasty flavor and fragrance.

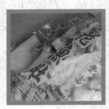

Fish Maw

Fish Maw is the air bladder of a large fish and is considered a delicacy. It is deep fried and available in dried form.

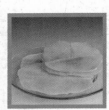

Dried Abalone

The properties of abalone were previously discussed (page 58). In its dried form it adds a tasty flavor to a soup.

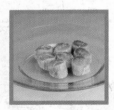

Dried Scallops

Dried Scallops have a much deeper taste and fragrance than fresh scallops. Several pieces in a pot of soup adds a sweet seafood taste.

Using Vegetables, Seeds and Fungi

The following is a short list of some vegetables typically used in traditional health soups. All are normally available from North American Asian markets and some are available from normal supermarkets.

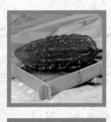

Bitter Melon (Bitter Gourd or Goya)

Bitter melon resembles a large cucumber with nodules on its surface. Bitter Melon has special health benefits, such as preventing colds and some illnesses and it also promotes digestion. Bitter Melon is *leung* (cooling) and has a slightly bitter taste. It is considered an important health food item.

Carrots

Carrots are considered as having neutral properties. They are moisturizing and soothing to the body and also contain Beta-carotene, an important source of vitamin A.

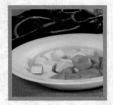

Garlic

Garlic has been used since ancient times by most cultures and is considered to have preventive properties against flu and many other problems. Garlic is frequently used in cooking Chinese dishes and vegetables. Garlic is considered *yit* (warming) and is added to green vegetables which are *leung* (cooling) to achieve *leung-yit* (cold and hot) balance.

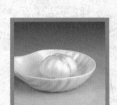

Napa (Brassica rapa)

Napa is mildly *leung* (cooling) cabbage. It is good for digestion and cleansing.

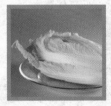

Lotus Root

Lotus Root is a water grown vegetable and as such is *leung* (cooling) and *yun* (moisturizing). It is used for making soup and is stir fried as a vegetable dish. It is very crunchy when just cooked and has a pleasant sweet taste.

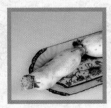

Watercress

Watercress also is a water grown vegetable. It is moisturizing and *leung* (cooling) as is evident by its distinct minty taste. It is used in both quick boiled and long boiled soups. It is also stir-fried with garlic as a vegetable dish and available in family style restaurants. This is a very good vegetable to balance a *yit* (hot) meal.

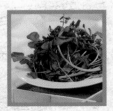

A Trip to the Chinese/Asian Market

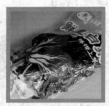

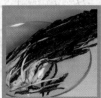

Cole (Dried Bok Choy)

Cole is used in one of the most common Chinese vegetable health soups. It is dark green and has *leung* (cooling) properties. Sun drying changes its flavor to a deep mellow taste. There are two types of cole, dark green and the light green. Both are equally beneficial. Generally, fresh bok choy is not used for health soups because it does not have the deep mellow flavor of cole. It is believed that sun drying enhances the *leung* (cooling) effect of cole and enhances its *yun* (moisturizing) abilities.

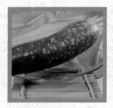

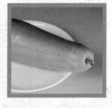

Fuzzy Squash and Opo Squash

Ded Gar comes in two main types, fuzzy (hairy) and opo (clear skin) squash. Both are slightly *leung* (cooling). They promote good digestion and elimination.

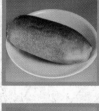

Green Lo Bok and White Lo Bok

Lo Bok (Chinese radish) comes in two types. Green lo bok is *leung* (cooling) as well as *yun* (moisturizing) and soothing. White lo bok is slightly *yit* (warming). Both provide beneficial plant based nutrients to the body and promote healing.

Winter Melon

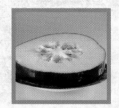

Winter Melon is naturally *leung* (cooling). Winter melon and especially its skin are used to alleviate skin problems and rashes. The skin of the winter melon is not removed when a very *leung* (cooling) soup is desired. The skin adds a deep flavor to the soup. Winter melon is thought to be good for bodily cleansing and toxin removal.

When used for healing purposes, the entire winter melon, including the pulp and seeds are often used.

Ginger

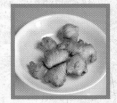

Ginger root is widely used in Chinese cooking both for its flavor as well as for its preventive properties. It is the classic *yit* (warming) ingredient that is used to counter balance *leung* (cooling) effects. Ginger is thought to strengthen the blood and to fight off minor infections and illnesses. When the body is weak, frail and suffering from a *leung* illness, ginger is used to stimulate internal heat (*yit*) and warm up the body. Elderly people or those frail in health often add ginger to *leung* (cooling) soups and vegetables to warm them up and achieve *leung-yit* (cold and hot) balance.

White Fungus (Snow Fungus)

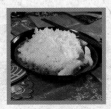

White or Snow Fungus (Tremella fuciformis) is a type of jelly mushroom. It is also sold under the name Weibe fungus. It is *leung* (cooling), moisturizing and cleansing.

Wolfberry (Giji, Guy Do, Lycium barbarum)

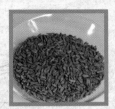

Wolfberry plants are often used as hedges. Wolfberry leaves are quick boiled with either pork or liver, making a nice broth that is reputed to be good for strengthening the eyes. Chinese believe that wolfberries contain many essential jing/essences that heal the body, particularly the blood and the eyes. Wolfberries are a popular health food item at health food stores.

A Trip to the Chinese/Asian Market

Traditonal Long Boiled (*Low For Tong*) Chinese Health Soups

Soup Index

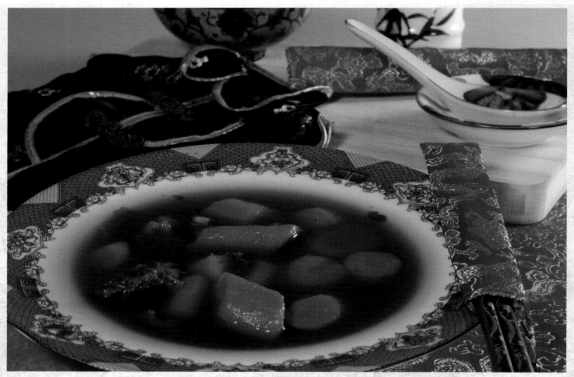

Chapter 6

Traditonal Long Boiled (*Low For Tong*)
Chinese Health Soups

Preparation Basics

This chapter presents recipes for traditional long boiled (*low for tong* -old fire) Chinese health soups. These soup recipes are favorites that have been passed from generation to generation.

Cooking Time

Hard ingredients such as beans, nuts, herbs and bones require a longer boiling time to extract and blend into the soup; while soft ingredients such as vegetables, seeds, thin pieces of meat require a shorter cooking time.

The cooking times for long boiled soups are based upon bringing the soup to an initial strong boil and then reducing the heat so that the soup gently simmers (bubbles) for a specified cooking time, normally 1 to 4 hours. During every hour of slow simmering, the liquid volume is reduced by about 8%. Conversely, increasing the boiling rate reduces the cooking time. When cooking at higher rates, do not cover to prevent boiling over.

Several other cooking options are also possible: After initial boiling, the cooking temperature can be lowered to 80 °C (175 °F) and the cooking time doubled; or the cooking temperature may be reduced to 65 °C (150 °F) and cooking time quadrupled. A slow cooker may also be used to make these soups. Start with boiling water and then set the slow cooker for about 14 to 16 hours at low heat, or 10 to 12 hours at medium heat. This will vary, depending on the individual slow cooker. We often start slow cook congees the night before and have them ready for breakfast. Or we start long boiled soup in the morning and have it for dinner.

Meat and Bones

Most of the listed soups have some meat and/or soup bones as base ingredients. Soups can become vegetarian soups by simply not adding any meat. Soups which have herbal ingredients normally require some meat, to take the edge off the herbal taste. Otherwise, the resulting stock may not be very palatable or tasty and could even cause irritation. A small amount of salt (5ml (1 tsp)) is normally added to all of these soups at the beginning of the cooking process to facilitate extraction of nutrients from the base ingredients. For many long-boiled soups, all solid ingredients that have been subject to the long cooking process are discarded after cooking; only the remaining liquid soup base is consumed. In seafood soups, the ingredients are normally consumed. For some soups, additional ingredients are added to the soup base at the end of the cooking process; these are consumed.

How To Make Long Boiled (*Low For Tong*) Soup

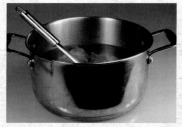 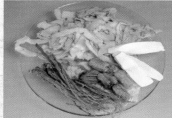 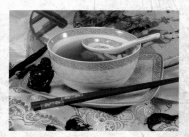

In A Nutshell

1. Blanch all meat and bones
2. Put all ingredients in a pot, add cold water covering 3 to 4 times the ingredient depth and add salt.

• Meat and bones used for soup are normally lower end cuts. Tough meats are often preferred because they have more flavor. I often cut off bones from pork chops or chicken and use for soup. Blanching will result in a much cleaner soup. If not blanched, skim off scum before serving. Lean chicken breast, pork chops or beef will result in a soup with less fat and grease.
• Soup ingredients constitute 20% to 30% of the contents in most long boiled soups. More meat will result in a sweeter and tastier soup. For those who wish to increase calcium in their diets, such as elderly people concerned about bone mass, adding bones to long boiled soup is an excellent way to add calcium to their diet. Tough meat such as oxtail, beef shank and pig knuckles require longer boiling times and are good for strengthening tendons, joints, and muscles.

3. Bring to a rapid boil for 2 min. Then lower the heat so that the soup just gently simmers for 1-4 hours, depending upon the soup. Check on the soup at regular intervals. Skim off all grease from the top of the pot. Taste the soup. If it is not salty enough, add salt to taste; if too salty, add boiling water. If the taste is still weak and undefined, cook for another hour. Once again, skim off any additional grease. The soup is now ready to serve. In long boiled soups, nutrients have been extracted into the broth and the ingredients are often discarded.

Blanching Meat

Blanching is the process of boiling meat and bones for a few minutes and then rinsing with cold water to get rid of grease and scum, resulting in a clearer soup.

1. Put meat or bones in a pot, add water to cover and bring to a boil. Continue boiling for a few minutes until color of the meat changes through the entire piece. Frozen meat and bones are cooked until completely thawed.

2. After blanching, pour into a large strainer and rinse with cold water until all scum is rinsed away. Cut away unwanted fat. The meat or bones are now ready for soup.

3. Fresh oxtail and beef are not normally blanched, as it may remove the sweet, natural flavor. However, if not very fresh, they should also be blanched.

Chicken Broth

Uses

Chicken broth is prepared as stock for soups and congees.

Ingredients

· 1 kg (2.2 lb) chicken or chicken bones
· Optional: Add lean pork to the broth. Although not necessary, the soup may taste sweeter. It is an accepted herbal practice to add pork to chicken soup to create a Yin Yang balance. Chicken is thought to be Yang and pork to be Yin.

Preparation

1. Blanch the chicken and remove any skin.
2. Place ingredients into a pot, adding 3.75 L (15 cups) cold water and 5 ml (1 tsp) salt. Bring to a rapid boil for 2 min. Then reduce the heat so that the soup just gently simmers. Maintain this rate of cooking for 1 to 2 hours.
3. Skim off all grease from the top of the pot. Taste the soup. If it is not salty enough add salt to taste; if too salty, add boiling water. If the taste still is weak and undefined, cook for another half hour. Once again, skim off any additional grease and remove and discard all solid ingredients, leaving only the liquid soup base.
4. Broth may be refrigerated for up to one week; alternately it can be frozen until used. Broth may also be prepared in a concentrated form and diluted upon use.

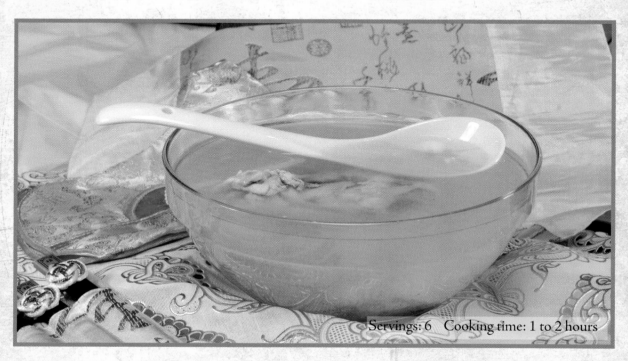

Servings: 6   Cooking time: 1 to 2 hours

Traditonal Long Boiled (*Low For Tong*) Chinese Health Soups

Cole and Carrot Soup

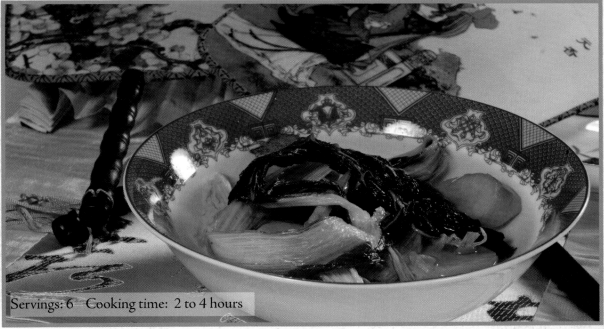

Servings: 6   Cooking time: 2 to 4 hours

Ingredients

- 1 bundle, 50 mm (2 in) diameter of cole (dried bok choy)
- 3 large carrots, peeled and sliced in 5 mm (0.2 in) long pieces
- 0.5 kg (1.1 lb) of either pork, beef, oxtail or duck (wing, neck, liver, kidneys and heart)
- Optional:
  - 2 - 4 honey dates
  - 1 clove dried mandarin or tangerine peels
  - 1 - 2 pieces (1 tbsp) of luo han guo fruit (siraitia grosvenori)

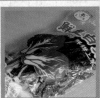

Preparation

1. Presoak the cole in warm water for 20 min or until fully hydrated and rinse.
2. Blanch meat.
3. Place the meat and all ingredients into a pot, adding 3.75 L (15 cups) cold water and 5 ml (1 tsp) salt. Bring to a rapid boil for 2 min. Then lower the heat so that the soup just gently simmers, for 4 hours. If oxtail, cooking time may have to be increased to 5-8 hours, depending on age of the oxtail. Skim off all grease from the top of the pot. Taste the soup. If it is not salty enough add salt to taste; if too salty, add boiling water. If the taste still is weak and undefined, cook for another hour.

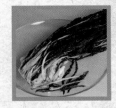

Health Properties

This is one of the most popular traditional health soups, used particularly during seasonal dryness. It is cooling, soothing and helps overcome dryness. It thought to have beneficial properties that moisten the lungs, assist with bodily cleansing, help healing and remove toxins. This soup is frequently used for treating sore throats, colds or flu.

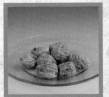

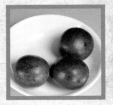

Traditonal Long Boiled (*Low For Tong*) Chinese Health Soups

Winter Melon Red Mung Bean Soup

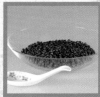

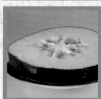

Ingredients

- 1 kg (2.2 lb) winter melon
- 125 ml (1/2 cup) to 250 ml (1 cup) red mung beans
- 0.5 kg (1.1 lb) pork or beef
- 3 large (40 mm (1.5 in) long) dried oysters

Note: If oxtail is used as the meat ingredient, cooking time may need to be increased up to 7 hours, depending on the age of the oxtail.

Preparation

1. Wash the winter melon in cold water. Cut off and discard the pulp in the centre as well as the seeds. Cut the winter melon into cubes about 40 mm (1.5 in) on each side. It is recommended to leave the skin on the melon as it adds nutritional value a well as enhancing the flavor. The green skin also provides *leung* (cooling) properties. Rinse mung beans in cold water.
2. Blanch meat.
3. Place all ingredients into pot, adding 3.75 L (15 cups) cold water and salt. Bring to a rapid boil for 2 min. Then lower the heat so that the soup just gently simmers for 4 hours. Skim off all grease.

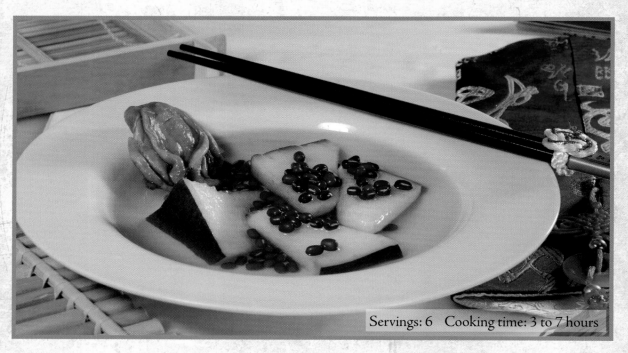

Servings: 6   Cooking time: 3 to 7 hours

Traditonal Long Boiled (*Low For Tong*) Chinese Health Soups

This classic soup is a great preventive soup. It is often served during illness. It is soothing and is believed to promote cleansing and recovery.

Being *leung yit* neutral, it is used to help the body regain balance from both extremes- *leung* (coldness) and *yit hay* (hot internal heat). Winter melon is cold like the winter. Its cooling properties are indicated by its green rind, snow white interior and cool taste. If used as a health tonic, the pulp and seeds may also be included in the soup, and are reputed to have extra cleansing and healing properties.

Red mung beans are thought to be good for detoxification, healing and cleansing. Red mung beans have a red exterior indicating slight *yit* (warming). Red mung beans offset the *leung* properties of the winter melon. The long boiling time blends the ingredients into a (*leung and yit*) neutral soup that helps the body balance itself. The long cooking process in itself warms and neutralizes the coldness of the winter melon. If the soup is boiled for only a short time, the soup will be *leung* (cold) from the winter melon as the warming properties have not yet neutralized the cooling properties. For people with excessive *leung*, the quantity of red mung beans may be increased to about 250 ml (1cup) and dried oysters may also be added to further counter the winter melon. This soup creates a soothing tonic that helps recovery from colds, flu and sore throats. It also helps reduce mucus and to revitalize the lungs. Winter Melon is also thought to cleanse the blood, treat skin problems, and help cleanse the body of toxins. This is one of the soups that I drink regularly to flush and cleanse my body of impurities.

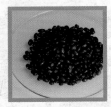

Small red mung (**Chick Sil Dow**) beans may be used instead of red mung beans. They are slightly smaller and a bit darker. Small red mung beans combined with winter melon (complete with skin, pulp and seeds) are used to treat skin conditions, especially red rash and red skin outbreaks.

Oyster is neutral and helps neutralize the cold properties of the winter melon. It is thought to be good for reducing fever, internal heat and perspiration. Oyster adds a pleasant seafood taste to the soup.

Winter Melon Green Mung Bean Soup

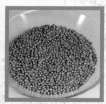

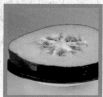

Ingredients
- 1 kg (2.2 lb) winter melon
- 125 ml (1/2 cup) to 250 ml (1 cup) green mung beans
- 0.5 kg (1.1 lb) pork, pork bones, beef, beef bones or oxtail
- 3 large (40 mm (1.5 in) long) dried oysters (optional).
- Note: If oxtail is used as the meat ingredient, cooking time may need to be increased up to 7 hours, depending on the age of the oxtail.

Preparation

1. Wash the winter melon in cold water. Cut off and discard the pulp in the center as well as the seeds. Seeds and pulp may also be used as they contain valuable healing nutrients. Cut the winter melon into cubes about 40 mm (1.5 in) on each side. It is recommended to leave the skin on the melon as it adds nutritional value and enhances the flavor as well. The green skin also provides *leung* (cooling) properties. Rinse mung beans in cold water.
2. Blanch meat.
3. Place all ingredients into pot, adding 3.75 L (15 cups) cold water and 5 ml (1 tsp) salt. Bring to a rapid boil for 2 min. Then lower the heat so that the soup just gently simmers for 4 hours or until the mung bean kernels are broken.
4. Skim off all grease.

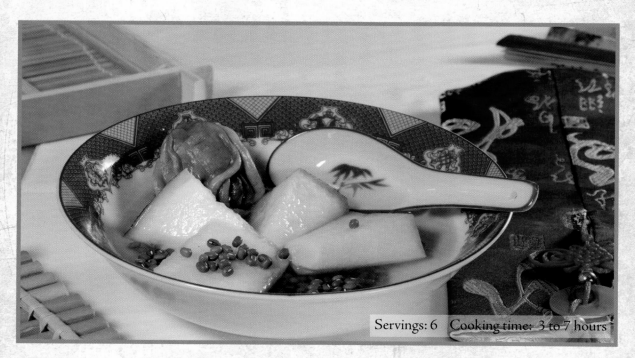

Servings: 6   Cooking time: 3 to 7 hours

Traditonal Long Boiled (*Low For Tong*) Chinese Health Soups

This is an everyday *leung* (cooling) soup and is good for *yit hay* (hot imbalance) illness. I drink this soup to help flush and cleanse impurities from my system. Being *leung* (cooling), it promotes urination and bowel movements. It is good for constipation and getting rid of fat and grease. This soup is often served during *yit hay* (excessive internal heat) type illnesses to provide *leung* (cooling) essences to counterbalance and help the body regain *leung-yit* (Yin Yang) balance. Winter Melon is also thought to cleanse the blood, treat skin problems, and help to cleanse the body of *yit doak* or hot toxins. Winter melon is cold like the winter. The green rind (skin), snow white interior and cold taste indicate that it is cooling. The green mung beans are considered to be very *leung* (cooling) while red mung beans are considered to be slightly *yit* (warming). This soup is good for *yit hay* (hot internal heat) related issues or just as a preventive health tonic.

Green mung beans are *leung* (cold) and are thought to be good for detoxication, cleansing and healing. Green mung beans are thought to be especially good for getting rid of *yit doak* (hot toxins).

The long cooking time combined with the meat and bones adds a warming element to the soup, making it less cold. It is important to boil the soup for at least four hours rendering it smooth, mellow and easy on the system. If the soup is boiled for only a short time, the soup will be very *leung* from the (cold) winter melon and (cold) green mung beans. The objective is to gently help the body balance itself and not to have a direct confrontation between *leung* and *yit* (hot and cold), which could aggravate matters.

For people with *yit hay* (excessive internal heat), the quantity of green mung beans should be increased to about 250 ml (1cup) to further the cooling and clearing properties. This soup creates a soothing tonic that helps recovery from colds, flu and sore throats. It also helps reduce yellow phlegm (mucus) and revitalizes the lungs. In case of white phlegm (mucus), use red mung beans instead.

Oyster is neutral and helps neutralize the cold properties of the winter melon and green mung beans. It is thought to be good for reducing fever, internal heat and perspiration. Oyster adds a pleasant seafood taste to the soup.

This soup is reputed to have very good cleansing properties, and helps the body get rid of mild toxins, especially *yit doak* (hot toxins). In order for this treatment to have an effect, a bowl of this soup should be consumed each day for two weeks. Mung beans are used to detoxify and are used in traditional Chinese medicine to treat mild poisoning. [17]

Black Turtle Bean Carrot Soup

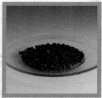

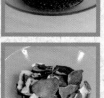

Ingredients

- 125 ml (0.5 cup) to 250 ml (1 cup) dried black turtle beans
- 3 large or 6 small carrots
- 0.7 kg (1.5 lb) beef or oxtail or pork
- 1 to 4 cloves of mandarin or tangerine peels

Preparation

1. Wash the turtle beans in cold water and drain.
2. If pork is used, blanch the meat. Trim fat from the meat. If beef or oxtail is used, pan fry for 3 to 5 minutes. (It is easier to buy pre-cut oxtail)
3. Put all ingredients in a pot, add 3.75 L (15 cups) water and salt. Bring to a rapid boil for 2 min. Then lower the heat so that the soup just gently simmers for 3 to 4 hours. If oxtail is used, cooking time may be increased up to 7 or 8 hours. Skim off all grease.

Health Properties

This classic soup tastes like consommé (beef broth). It reputedly helps to strengthen the *qi* (breathing) ability and is *leung* (cooling). This soup is nutritious and is especially good for people who eat little or no meat. Oxtail is tasty and is consumed. Oxtail is good for strengthening bones, joints, tendons and building blood. It is also good for building energy when you are weak and tired. Mandarin peels are good for clearing the lungs, reducing coughs and phlegm (mucous). Black turtle beans are *leung* (cooling) but may be pan fried to neutralize this property.

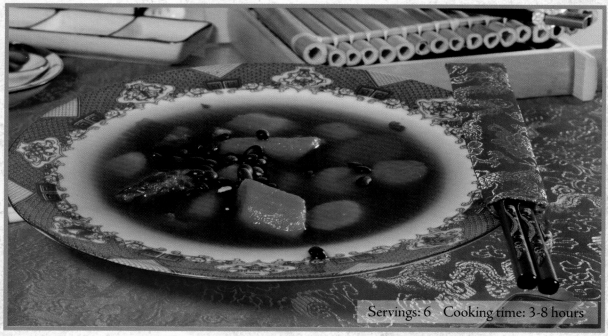

Servings: 6   Cooking time: 3-8 hours

Traditonal Long Boiled (*Low For Tong*) Chinese Health Soups

76

Green Lo Bok with Black Turtle Bean Soup

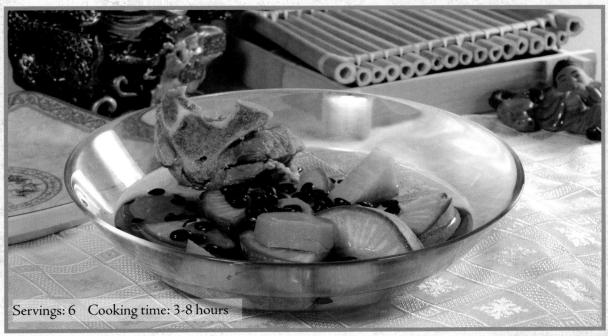

Servings: 6   Cooking time: 3-8 hours

Ingredients

- 0.5 kg (1.1 lb) green lo bok (Chinese radish)
- 125ml (0.5 cup) to 250 ml (1 cup) dried black turtle beans
- 0.5 kg (1.1 lb) beef or oxtail, or pork
- 2 to 4 carrots (optional)
- 1 to 4 cloves of mandarin or tangerine peels

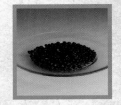

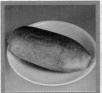

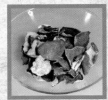

Preparation

1. Wash black turtle beans, lo bok and carrots. Peel and cut lo bok into chunks.

2. If pork is used, blanch the meat. If beef or oxtail is used, pan fry for 3 to 5 minutes. (It is easiest to buy pre-cut oxtail)

3. Put all ingredients in pot add 3.75 L (15 cups) water and salt. Bring to a rapid boil for 2 min. Then lower the heat so that the soup just gently simmers for 3 to 4 hours. If oxtail is used, cooking time may be increased up to 7 or 8 hours. Skim off all grease.

Health Properties

This classic Chinese home-style soup tastes a bit like consommé (beef broth). It strengthens the *qi* (breathing) ability. It is *leung* (cooling) and moisturizing. Green lo bok is *leung* (cooling), while white lo bok is *yit* (warming). Black turtle beans are *leung* (cooling) but may be pan fried to neutralize. Carrots are *yun* or moisturizing. Mandarin peels are good for clearing the lungs, reducing coughs and phlegm (mucous). The oxtail is tasty and is normally consumed. The oxtail is good for building blood, strengthening tendons, joints, bones and muscles. This soup is nutritious and is especially good for building physical energy. This soothing soup is often served when ill.

Traditonal Long Boiled (*Low For Tong*) Chinese Health Soups

Lotus Root Squid Soup

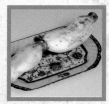

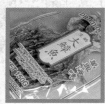

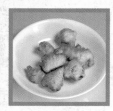

Ingredients

- 0.5 kg (1.1 lb) to 0.75 kg (1.7 lb) fresh lotus root or 0.23 kg (0.5 lb) dried lotus root
- 1 piece ginger, 2.5 cm (1 in) cube, or more for a *Yit* (warming) soup
- 0.5 kg (1.1 lb) pork or pork bones
- 1 piece of dried squid or dried octopus

Preparation

1. Blanch the meat and bones.
2. Cut the lotus root into individual links. Cut and discard all connective tissue between the links. Peel the links, cut into bite sized pieces and wash in cold water.
3. Place all ingredients in pot, add 3.75 L (15 cups) cold water; add salt. Bring to a rapid boil for 2 min. Then lower the heat so that the soup just gently simmers for 4 hours. Skim off all fat.

Health Properties

This tasty soup has a seafood flavor from the squid or octopus, blended with the sweet mellow taste of lotus root mixed in with a hint of ginger. Lotus root is *leung* (cooling) and when simmered for several hours it becomes mellow as it changes from off-white to pink. Ginger is added to neutralize the *leung* (cooling) effect, making the soup more neutral. If you want the soup to be *leung* (cooling), do not add any ginger. If you want the soup to be *yit* (warming), increase the amount of ginger. The lotus root is moisturizing and helps to prevent coughs. This soup is soothing and moisturizing.

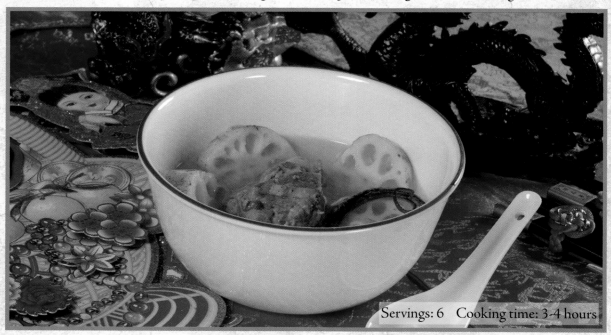

Servings: 6   Cooking time: 3-4 hours

Traditonal Long Boiled (*Low For Tong*) Chinese Health Soups

White Lo Bok Star Aniseed Soup

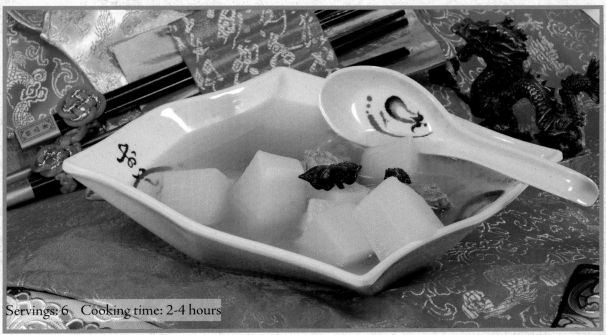

Servings: 6   Cooking time: 2-4 hours

Ingredients

- 1 kg (2.2 lb) white lo bok (white Chinese radish)
- 25 ml (1.5 tbsp - 2 to 4 pieces) dried star aniseed (Anise)
- 0.5 kg (1.1 lb) to 1 kg (2.2 lb) beef, or pork
- Optional: 2 to 4 sliced carrots

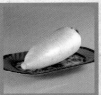

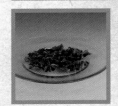

Preparation

1. If pork is used, blanch the meat and the bones.
2. If beef is used, stir fry for 3 to 5 min.
3. Peel lo bok and cut into bite sized pieces.
4. Place all ingredients in pot with 3.75 L (15 cups) water and salt. Bring to a rapid boil for 2 min, lower the heat so that the soup just gently simmers for 2 to 4 hours. Skim off all fat.

Health Properties

This is an everyday soup with a different taste that may take a while to appreciate. The soup is warming, promoting digestion and circulation. It is especially good during cold weather. Star aniseeds have a pungent taste, and are *yit* (warming). Star aniseeds contain shikimic acid, a primary feedstock used to create a popular anti-flu drug. For soups, buy only food grade star aniseed from reputable stores.

Arrowroot Sugarcane Soup

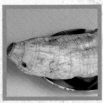

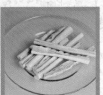

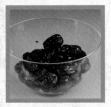

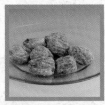

Ingredients

- 0.5 to 1 kg (1.1 to 2.2 lb) pork, pork bones or chicken
- One arrowroot 1 to 2 kg (2.2 to 4.4 lb), peeled and sliced into bite sized pieces

Any or all of :

- 4 to10 pieces fresh or dried sugarcane 10 cm (4 in) long
- 3 to 6 large honey dates
- 4 to 8 dried red dates
- 2 to 4 large carrots, washed and sliced

Preparation

1. Blanch the meat and bones.
2. Put ingredients in a pot adding 3.75 L (15 cups) cold water and 5 ml (1 tsp) salt. Bring to a rapid boil for 2 min. Then lower the heat so that the soup just gently simmers. Let the soup simmer for 4 to 8 hours. Discard all solids and skim off all fat, leaving only the soup broth.

Health Properties

This sweet soothing soup is *yun* (moisturizing) and *leung* (cooling). This soup is reputedly beneficial for reducing bad cholesterol and *yit hay* (hot) imbalance. This soup also has jing/essences beneficial for *yun fay* (moisturizing the lungs), reducing dryness and coughing. This lubricating soup is excellent during seasonal dryness.

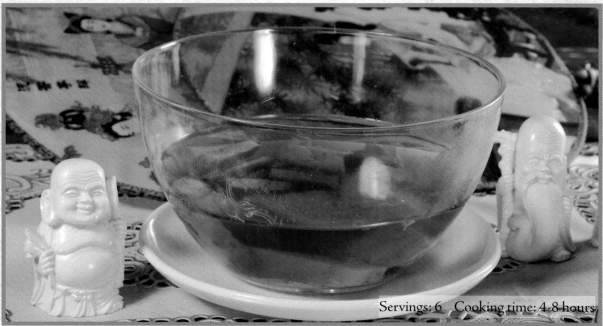

Servings: 6   Cooking time: 4-8 hours

Vegetable Soup

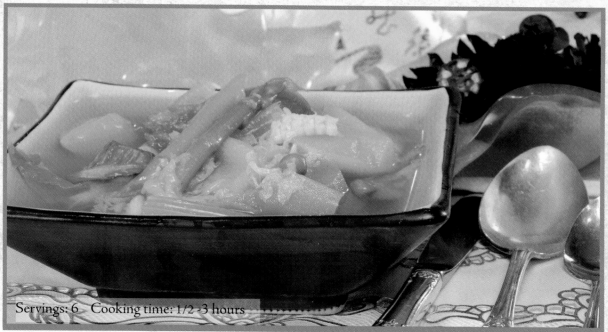

Servings: 6   Cooking time: 1/2 -3 hours

This soup can be short boiled (20 -30 minutes), or long boiled 1 to 3 hours. If short boiled the ingredients are consumed. When long boiled, valuable nutrients are extracted and may be consumed as a broth. When long boiled Lima beans, red or white kidney beans, black turtle beans, black-eyed peas and barley may be added, especially if meat is not used.

Ingredients

Use seasonally available vegetables in portions of preference. I prefer having a large quantity of rutabaga and carrots in this soup. Vegetables are peeled, sliced and washed. Vegetables used include: carrots, rutabaga, potatoes, cabbage, napa, onions, celery, peppers, broccoli stems, tomatoes, peas, corn and lo bok.

- 0.5 to 1 kg (1.1 to 2.2 lb) beef, pork or chicken. Trim fat from the meat.
- If beef is used, stir fry for 3 to 5 min. Add some light soy sauce (optional).

Preparation

1. Add prepared vegetables and about 3.75 L (15 cups) cold water, covering all ingredients to at least 2 times their depth. The ratio of water to ingredients will determine if the soup is chunky or light. Add salt together with seasoning such as fine herbs and oregano, if desired. Bring to a rapid boil for 2 min. Lower heat so that the soup gently simmers for ½ to 2 hours. Skim off all grease from the top of the pot.

Herbal Variation: Add 15 to 45 ml (1 to 3 tbsp) of wolfberries; this will make the soup taste sweet.

Health Properties

Vegetables and beans contain many nutrients essential to good health. This soup provides a rainbow of valuable healing nutrients needed for good health and is especially useful for those suffering a weakening illness and those who are unable to eat solid food. Vegetable soup is yun (moisturizing) and leung (cooling), cleansing, promoting urination and bowel movement. Beans provide additional valuable jing/essences essential to healing and rebuilding. Wolfberry is thought to be beneficial to the eyes and increases sperm count. Wolfberry contains beta-carotene and jing/essences that are reputed to build up resistance and to strengthen the body.

Traditonal Long Boiled (*Low For Tong*) Chinese Health Soups

Bean Curd Stick Seafood Soup

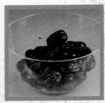

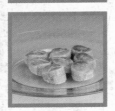

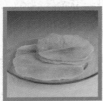

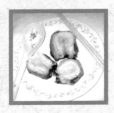

Ingredients

- 3 to 6 pieces of dried scallops
- 15 ml (1 tbsp) dried shrimp
- 2 to 5 large (4.0 cm (1.5 in) long) dried oysters
- 28 g (1 oz) dried black fungus (black hair fungus)
- 170 g (6 oz) dried bean curd stick
- 2 large dried Shitake (black) mushroom soaked to soften and then sliced
- 0.9 kg (2 lb) chicken and/or pork, or pig knuckles
- **Optional Ingredients**
- 140 g (5 oz) canned clams
- 4 to 8 Chinese red dates
- 3 to 6 peeled and sliced fresh water chestnuts
- Abalone (see below)

Preparation

1. Blanch meat and bones.
2. Place all ingredients except the dried bean curd in 3.75 L (15 cups) cold water. Add salt. Bring to a rapid boil for 2 min. Then lower the heat so that the soup just gently simmers for 3 to 4 hours.
3. Break the dried bean curd sticks into 8.0 cm (3 in) long pieces and soak in cold water for about 20 min, until soft. Shortly before serving, add the bean curd to the soup broth, bring to a full boil and simmer for 10 min. The soup is now ready to serve.

Abalone:

• If it is sliced, use 3 to 5 slices

• If dried whole, abalone must be soaked in cold water for about 24 hours to soften, before slicing.

• If fresh frozen, use 0.2 kg (0.5 lb), thaw, boil in water for 5 min, rinse in cold water, scrape off the black outer layer, and cut into bite-sized pieces before adding to the soup.

• If canned, use one 425 g (15 oz) can, slicing the abalone into about 5 mm (0.2 in) thick slices. Add abalone with juice 10 minutes before serving. Do not overcook as it will become rubbery.

Warning: Those with heart problems are advised not to eat abalone.

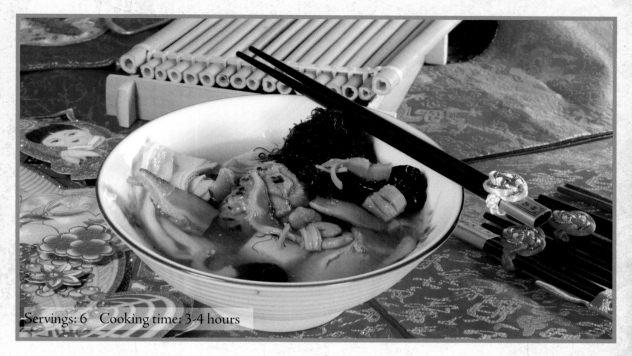

Servings: 6   Cooking time: 3-4 hours

Health Properties

This tasty seafood soup is a Chinese celebration soup. Hair fungus - *Fat Choy* sounds like "get rich" in Chinese. Often served at New Years, it is a favorite among seafood lovers. Seafood contains nutrients that are beneficial to the body, especially the kidneys and the bladder. Abalone is good for strengthening the bladder and is used to control urination. Bean curd is *leung* (cooling) and is good for reducing *yit hay* (hot internal heat). Bean curd is reputedly good for removing water from body, promoting urination and improving blood circulation. Hair fungus is reputed to cleanse the intestines. Red dates (jujube) have soothing healing sugars, are good for the blood and are thought to have preventive properties. In Chinese culture, red dates and walnuts are placed in newly weds' bedrooms as a sign of fertility. In this soup, the red dates add a cheerful red to the soup, indicating happiness. Red dates are referred to as nature's vitamin pill because they contain an array of vitamins.

Traditonal Long Boiled (*Low For Tong*) Chinese Health Soups

White Fungus Soup

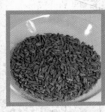

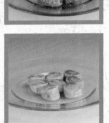

Ingredients

- 2 to 3 dried white (snow) fungus, each 7.5 cm (3 in) diameter
- 0.9 kg (2 lb) chicken and/or pork
- 15 to 45 ml (1 to 3 tbsp) wolfberries

Optional Ingredients

- 2 to 4 honey dates
- 5 to 10 pieces of Solomon's Seal (polygonatum)
- 2 to 5 pieces dried scallops, 2.5 cm (1 in) diameter.

Preparation

1. Soak the white fungus in warm water for 20 min, until soft. Discard the central dark yellow stems and cut the leafy parts into bite size pieces.
2. Blanch the meat.
3. Place all ingredients, except the white fungus in a large pot, adding 3.75 L (15 cups) cold water and 5 ml (1tsp) salt. Bring to a rapid boil for 2 min then reduce heat to a gentle simmer for 2 to 4 hours.
4. Skim off all fat.
5. Add the white fungus to the soup broth, bring to a boil and simmer for 10 to 30 min. The soup is now ready to serve. The white fungus may be eaten. (Do not overcook. White fungus may become jelly-like if overcooked.)

Health Properties

This soup has both moisturizing and cleansing properties. White fungus (also known as snow fungus or Weibe fungus) is very popular in Chinese cuisine. It is reputed to have many preventive health properties and is thought to be especially good for the heart and lungs. It is cooling and is thought to be *yun fay* (moisturize the lungs). Wolfberries are thought to be good for strengthening the eyes, increasing sperm count and helping the body rebuild and heal.

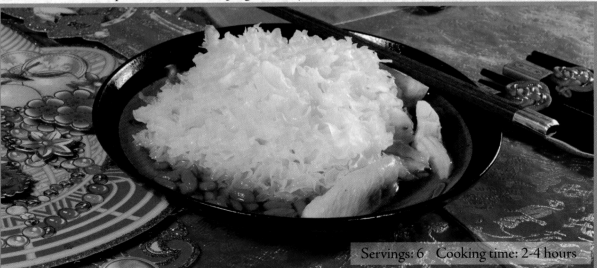

Servings: 6   Cooking time: 2-4 hours

Traditonal Long Boiled (*Low For Tong*) Chinese Health Soups

Black-Eyed Pea Carrot Soup

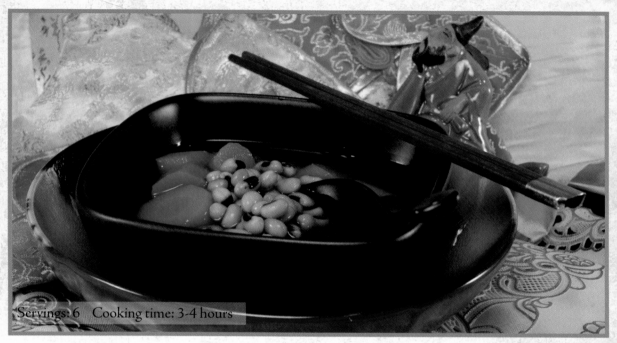

Servings: 6   Cooking time: 3-4 hours

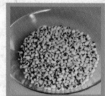

Ingredients

- 250 to 500 ml (1 to 2 cups) dried black-eyed peas
- 0.9 kg (2 lb) pork, pork bones and/or chicken
- 2 large or 4 small carrots

Preparation

1. Blanch the meat and bones.
2. Peel and wash the carrots, cutting them into bite-size pieces.
Rinse the black-eyed peas in cold water and drain.
3. Place the meat and all ingredients into a large pot, adding 3.75 L (15 cups) cold water and 5 ml (1 tsp) salt. Bring to a rapid boil for 2 minutes, then reduce heat to a gentle simmer for 3 to 4 hours.
4. Skim off all fat. Remove and discard any meat and bones, leaving only the liquid broth with peas and carrots. The soup is now ready to serve.

Health Properties

This soup is thought to be good for the lungs. Blacked-eyed peas are believed to strengthen the *qi* (breathing). Carrots are a good source of beta-carotene, which the body converts to Vitamin A. Carrots are good for the eyes and are *yun* (moisturizing).

Oxtail Stew

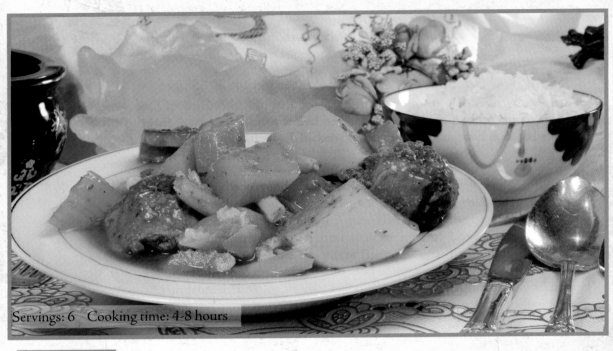

Servings: 6   Cooking time: 4-8 hours

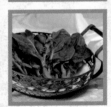

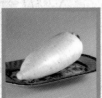

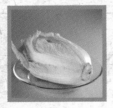

Ingredients

Oxtail stew, similar to a chunky soup, contains an abundantly thick sauce and is served over a bed of rice. Use seasonally available vegetables such as: carrots, rutabaga, potatoes, cabbage, onions, celery, peppers, broccoli stems, tomatoes, peas and corn. To make it a distinctively Chinese stew, add napa, lo bok and Chinese broccoli. Oxtail stew may require increased cooking time, up to 8 hours, depending on the age of the oxtail. The first group of vegetables will breakdown and become soggy while some will become sauce, so consider adding more vegetables later, about 45 minutes before serving. It is great over a bed of rice.

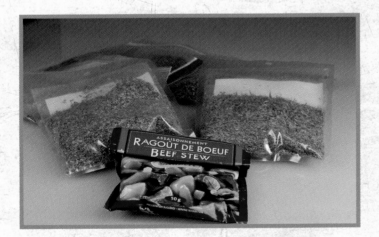

Traditonal Long Boiled (*Low For Tong*) Chinese Health Soups

Preparation

1. Peel, cut and wash vegetables.
2. Trim fat from 1.5 kg (3.3 lb) of pre-cut oxtail.
3. Stir fry the oxtail in the pot for 3 to 5 min, adding light soy sauce if desired.
4. Add prepared vegetables and water, covering all ingredients with at least 2.5cm (1 in) of water. Add salt together with seasoning such as fine herbs, oregano, and stew seasoning. Bring to a rapid boil for 2 min. Lower heat so that the stew gently simmers for 2 to 5 hours. Skim off all grease.
5. Add the remainder of the vegetables about 45 minutes before serving. Add boiling water, if necessary, to cover all ingredients.
6. Optional: Thicken the broth by adding 15ml (1 tbsp) of corn starch or tapioca flour mixed in 60ml (0.25 cups) of cold water, then slowly blend the slurry into the hot stew. Repeat until thickened to the desired degree, adding boiling water if it becomes too thick.

Variation

To also have some crunchy vegetables, set aside some vegetables until the stew is almost ready. Add any of the following which cook quickly: broccoli, Chinese broccoli, tomatoes, peppers, celery, cabbage, napa or cauliflower and boil for 1 to 5 min, depending how crunchy you prefer the vegetables.

Health Properties

This is a comfort food that nourishes the body and calms the soul. It is a complete and balanced meal that is great on a cold day. The long boiling process extracts the meat and plant nutrients into the sauce so that they are easily absorbed by the body. Mushy vegetables are easy to digest and may increase the frequency of bowel movements, helping to cleanse the body. Stew is a great meal for those who are suffering from illness and for elderly people. Oxtail is good for building and strengthening tendons, joints, muscles, and enhancing physical energy.

Chinese Style Beef Stew with Rice

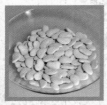

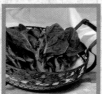

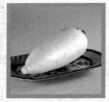

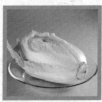

Ingredients

This Chinese version of beef stew is similar to a chunky soup because it contains a thick sauce and is served over a bed of rice. Use seasonally available vegetables such as: carrots, rutabaga, potatoes, cabbage, onions, celery, peppers, broccoli stems, tomatoes, peas and corn. To make it a distinctively Chinese stew, add napa, lo bok and Chinese broccoli. If vegetarian -Lima beans and/or kidney beans may be added for protein.

Preparation

1. Peel, cut and wash vegetables.
2. Trim fat from 1.5 kg (3.3 lb) to 2 kg (4.4 lb) beef and cut into 25 cm (1 in) cubes.
3. Stir fry beef for 3 to 5 min. in the pot, adding light soy sauce if desired.
4. Add prepared vegetables and water, covering all ingredients to a depth of at least 2.5 cm (1 in). Add salt together with seasoning such as fine herbs, oregano, and stew seasoning. Bring to a rapid boil for 2 min. Lower heat so that the stew gently simmers for 1 to 3 hours. Skim off all grease.
5. Optional: Thicken the broth by adding 15 ml (1 tbsp) of corn starch or tapioca flour mixed in 60 ml (0.25 cups) of cold water; then slowly blend slurry into the hot stew. Repeat until thickened to the desired degree, adding boiling water if is too thick.

Variation

To have some crunchy vegetables, set aside some vegetables until the stew is almost ready. Add any of the following which cook quickly: broccoli, Chinese broccoli, tomatoes, peppers, celery, cabbage, napa or cauliflower and boil for 1 to 5 min depending how crunchy you like the vegetables.

Note: Once the stew is starched, do not reheat at a high temperature as the bottom will burn. To avoid this problem consider reheating in a microwave.

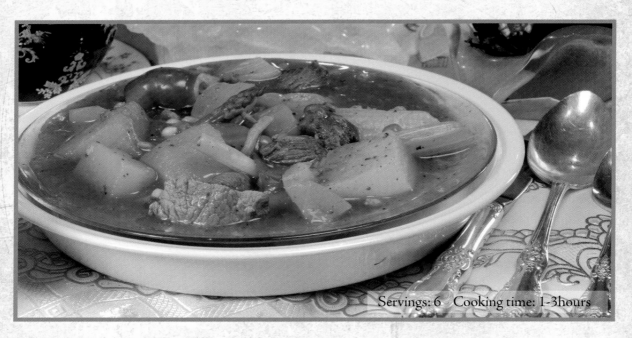

Servings: 6   Cooking time: 1-3hours

Traditonal Long Boiled (*Low For Tong*) Chinese Health Soups

88

Watercress Soup

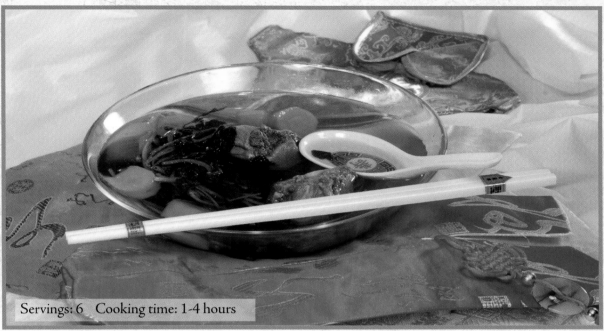

Servings: 6   Cooking time: 1-4 hours

Ingredients

- 2 bundles watercress, 75 mm (3 in) diameter by 100 mm (4 in) long
- 0.5 kg (1.1 lb) chicken, pork, beef, or oxtail

Optional Ingredients:

- 2 large or 4 small carrots
- 125 ml (0.5 cup) washed black turtle beans
- 30 ml (2 tbsp) almonds or apricot pits
- 3 large honey dates

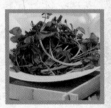

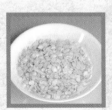

Preparation

1. Soak and wash the watercress three times until all the debris is removed.
2. Blanch the meat.
3. Put ingredients into a pot. Add salt and 2.5 L (10 cups) cold water. Bring to a rapid boil for 2 min. Then lower heat so soup just gently simmers for 1 to 4 hours. Skim off the grease.

Health Properties

This is one of the most popular Chinese health soups. The pleasant minty taste of watercress indicates that it is *leung* (cooling). It is used to prevent or offset *yit hay* (hot) imbalance. When cooked for several hours, the taste mellows and the watercress becomes neutral and soothing. The honey dates and carrots are sweet and moisturizing. This is an everyday soup which is used to help relieve dryness and dry coughs. Almonds or apricot pits are added to relieve upper chest congestion, reduce phlegm (mucous), ease breathing and lubricate the intestines. Watercress soup is *leung* (cooling), moisturizing and soothing and good for colds and flu. It reputedly cleanses hot (*yit*, Yang) toxins from the body to maintain an appropriate *leung yit* (cold hot) internal balance.

Traditional Chinese Health Tonic/Soups

Soup Index

	Possible Soup Broths				Page
	chicken	pork	beef	vegetarien	
Ginger Beef Tonic			✦		92
Ginger Chicken Tonic	✦				93
American Ginseng Herbal Tonic	✦	✦		✦	94
American Ginseng Tonic				✦	95
Liver Wolfberry Tonic	✦	✦			96
Sugarcane Carrot Tonic	✦	✦	✦	✦	97
Salty Arrowroot Paste				✦	98
Abalone or Conch Chicken Soup	✦	✦			99

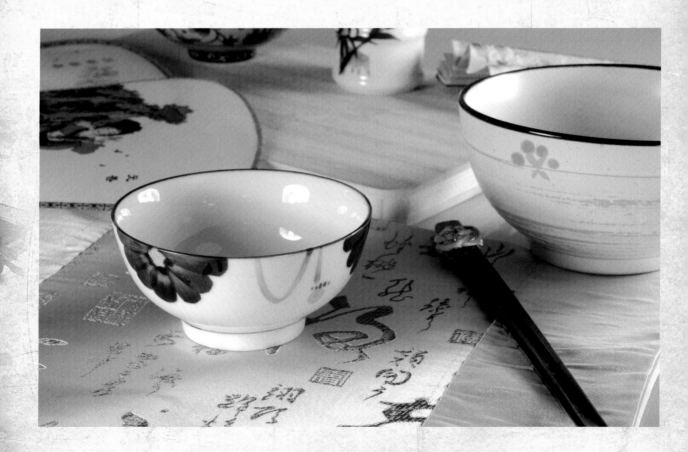

Chapter 7

Traditional Chinese Health Tonic/Soups

The Basics

Traditional Chinese medicine believes that premature aging and illness are the result of an imbalanced diet and lifestyle. It is further believed that some illnesses are caused by shortages of essential jing/essences, internal energy deficiencies, imbalances and dryness. However, if the body is kept in balance and not overwhelmed by unhealthy excesses, it will stay healthy and may slow its aging. A major way to prevent serious illness is to drink appropriate long boiled health soups containing powerful plant phytochemicals that heal.

Key objectives of soups are to:

· Strengthen the body with jing/essences .
· *Yit* or warm up the internal energy with Yang (hot) food.
· *Leung* or cool down the internal energy with Yin (cool) food.
· Help the body to achieve *leung yit* (Yin Yang) equilibrium.
· Supply the body with required *Yun fay* (moisturizing) essences.
· Foster cleansing and prevent buildup of *Yit doak* (hot) toxins.

Ginger Beef Tonic

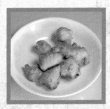

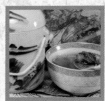

Ingredients
- Several 5 mm (0.25 in) thick slices of fresh ginger
- 0.25 to 0.5 kg (0.6 to 1.1 lb) beef chunks or beef shank, with fat trimmed off
- Pinch of salt

Preparation

1. **Double Boiler Method:** To extract maximum nutrients use a double boiler (left) which lets you cook over (not in) boiling water. Fill the bottom bowl three quarters full with boiling water. Place all ingredients in the top bowl and fill it with boiling water to the same level. Insert the top bowl into the bottom bowl. Bring the bottom bowl to a boil and reduce to a gentle simmer for 2 to 4 hours. Add boiling water, as required, every 30 minutes. Discard the solid ingredients and enjoy the tonic.

2. **Regular Method:** Put all ingredients into a pot, adding 1 L (4 cups) cold water. Bring to a rapid boil for 2 min. Then lower the heat so that the soup just gently simmers for 2 to 4 hours. Skim off all fat. Discard the solid ingredients and enjoy the tonic

Health Properties

This tonic increases body energy, enhances resistance to illness and is good for those suffering weaknesses. Beef is a good source of protein, builds muscles and is thought to increase endurance and stamina. Ginger is *yit* (hot), warms the body and is used to combat a *leung* (cold) conditions. Vary the amount of ginger to taste. For *yit hay* (hot) internal energy imbalance, use little or no ginger. For *leung* (cold) internal energy imbalance, increase the ginger. Ginger reputedly helps to build blood and is good for physical weakness and exhaustion. It is used for illness recovery and prevention. This tonic is beneficial to those who cannot eat solid food or who lack meat in their diet.

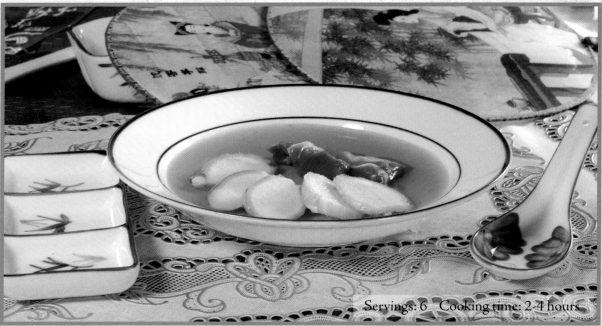

Servings: 6   Cooking time: 2-4 hours

(Ginger and beef shown before cooking)

Ginger Chicken Tonic

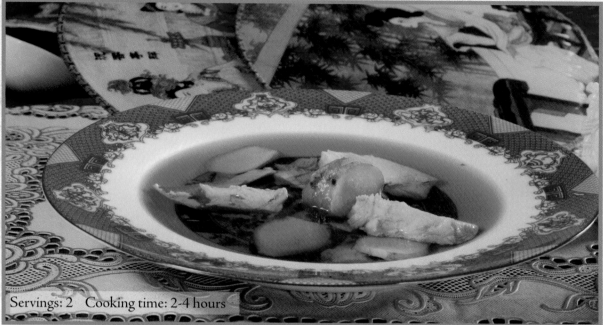

Servings: 2   Cooking time: 2-4 hours

Ingredients

- 0.25 to 0.5 kg (0.6 to 1.1 lbs) chicken, skinned with fat removed and cut into pieces
- Several 5 mm (0.25 in) thick slices of fresh ginger
- Pinch of salt

Preparation

1. Double Boiler Method: To extract maximum nutrients use a double boiler (right) which lets you cook over (not in) boiling water. Fill the bottom bowl three quarters full with boiling water. Place all ingredients in the top bowl and fill it with boiling water to the same level. Insert the top bowl into the bottom bowl. Bring the bottom bowl to a boil and reduce to a gentle simmer for 2 to 4 hours. Add boiling water, as required, every 30 minutes.

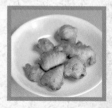

2. Regular Method: Blanch chicken and put all ingredients into a pot, adding 1 L (4 cups) cold water. Bring to a rapid boil for 2 min. Then lower the heat so that the soup just gently simmers for 2 to 4 hours. Skim off all fat.

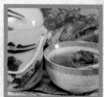

Health Properties

This tonic increases body energy and enhances resistance to illness. Chicken soup is acclaimed for relieving symptoms of colds and flu. Chicken soup is good for physical weakness and exhaustion. Ginger being *yit* (hot), warms the body and is used to combat a *leung* (cold) condition. Vary the amount of ginger to taste. For *yit hay* (hot) internal energy imbalance, use little or no ginger. For *leung* (cold) internal energy imbalance, increase the ginger. This tonic is beneficial for those who cannot eat solid food or who lack meat in their diet.

American Ginseng Herbal Tonic

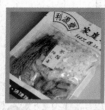

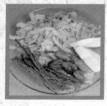

Ingredients

- Small, thin, American ginseng roots; honey dates; yam (dioscorea), Solomon's seal (polygonatium). This soup mix is available in pre-packaged format (left).
- 1 kg (2.2 lb) chicken
- Optional: 0.25 kg (0.5 lb) pork

Preparation

1. Blanch meat and bones.
2. Put all ingredients in pot adding 4 L (16 cups) cold water and 5 ml (1 tsp) salt. Bring to a rapid boil for 2 min. Then lower the heat so that the soup just gently simmers for 1 ½ to 3 hours. Discard all solids and skim off all fat, leaving only the tonic. If it is too strong or bitter, add boiling water.

Health Properties

This tonic has a minty herbal taste that is believed to help get rid of *yit doak* (hot toxins). It is quite *leung* (cooling), *yun* (moisturizing), and soothing. American ginseng has a minty taste, is renowned for its *leung* (cooling) qualities and is good for preventing *yit hay* (hot) imbalance. Chicken makes the soup mellow and takes the edge off the American ginseng. Honey dates, yam and Solomon's seal are soothing, moisturizing and help reduce dryness. This tonic is especially good during seasonal dryness. Being quite *leung*, it promotes urination and bowel movement. This tonic helps the body cleanse itself, and is ideal for balancing a diet. It is used to counteract *yit hay* (hot) food. *Herbalists normally advise not consuming any ginseng when ill*, to avoid direct confrontation between extreme hot and cold which may cause an adverse reaction. Wait until the illness is completely over. Novices should drink very little of this the first time and gage its effect. Ginseng is a widely used food supplement. If you have any doubt, consult a trained herbalist or doctor beforehand to avoid any side effects.

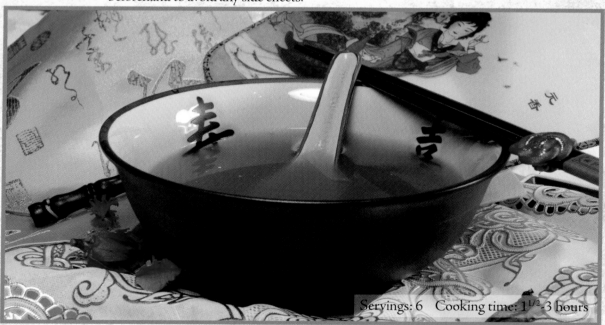

Servings: 6   Cooking time: 1½-3 hours

American Ginseng Tonic

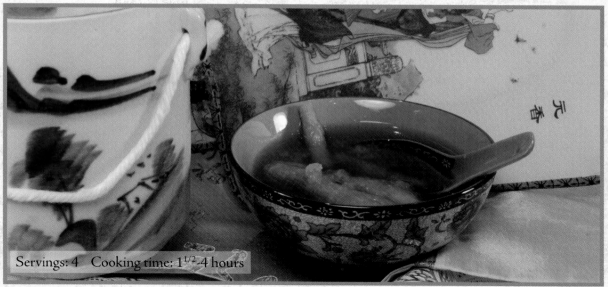

Servings: 4   Cooking time: 1$^{1/2}$-4 hours

Ingredients

+ 2 or 3 large American ginseng roots, 15 mm (0.5 in) diameter
+ 15 to 30 ml (1 to 2 tbsp) rice
+ Pinch of salt

Preparation

1. Double Boiler Method: To extract maximum nutrients use a double boiler (above) which lets you cook over (not in) boiling water. Fill the bottom bowl three quarters full with boiling water. Place all ingredients in the top bowl and fill it with boiling water to the same level. Insert the top bowl into the bottom bowl. Bring the bottom bowl to a boil and reduce to a gentle simmer for 2 to 4 hours. Add boiling water, as required, every 30 minutes.

2. Regular Method: Put all ingredients in pot adding 1.5 L (6 cups) cold water and bring to a rapid boil for 2 min. Then lower the heat so that the soup just gently simmers for 1 ½ to 4 hours. Discard all solids, leaving only the tonic.

Note: Do not confuse American ginseng with Korean ginseng. American ginseng is white inside while Korean ginseng is larger, heavier, dark reddish inside and is an energy tonic.

Health Properties

When the Chinese came to North America to build railroads in the 1800's, they discovered this minty herb that characterizes the coldness of a cold land. North American ginseng is more valued than that grown elsewhere. This tonic has a strong minty herbal taste and reputedly helps get rid of *yit doak* (hot toxins). It may be served hot or cold. It is strong and only 125 to 250 ml (0.5 to 1 cup) should be consumed daily. If it is too strong or bitter, dilute with boiling water. Rice is used to take the edge off the herb, is very *leung* (cold) and is used for preventive purposes only. This tonic helps to moisturize and reduce internal dryness, especially during seasonal dryness. It cleanses and promotes urination and bowel movement. *Herbalists normally advise not consuming any ginseng when ill*, to avoid direct confrontation between extreme hot and cold which may cause an adverse reaction. Wait until the illness is completely over. Novices should drink very little of this the first time and gage its effect. Ginseng is considered a food supplement. If you have any doubt, consult a trained herbalist or doctor beforehand to avoid any side effects.

Liver Wolfberry Tonic

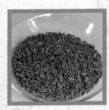

Ingredients
- 0.5 kg (1.1 lb) pork liver
- 30 to 90 ml (2 to 6 tbsp) of dried wolfberry (Giji, Guy Do, Lycium barbarum), more or less
- Salt to taste

Preparation
1. Rinse ingredients
2. Put all ingredients in pot and add 1L (4 cups) cold water. Bring to a rapid boil for 2 min. Then lower the heat so that the soup just gently simmers for 2 to 4 hours. Discard all solids and enjoy the tonic.

Health Properties
The Chinese believe there is a Yin Yang relationship between the liver and the eyes. When you have jaundice, the eyes become yellow. In preventing eye problems, both the eyes and the liver must be treated. This tonic is an ancient Chinese herbal recipe for strengthening the eyes and treating eye problems. It warms the internal energy and is used to increase strength. While it may not heal serious eye problems, it may help reduce deterioration.

Wolfberry is a popular health food item in many cultures and is quickly being adopted in Western culture as a health food snack item. Chinese herbalists have long used wolfberries for their many healing properties and believe they are best in soups or tonics. Wolfberry is orange in color indicating a high concentration of beta-carotene and is used to strengthen the eyes, build blood, to increase physical energy and enhance endurance. Wolfberry is believed to contain jing/essences that help strengthen and repair the body, and increase sperm count.

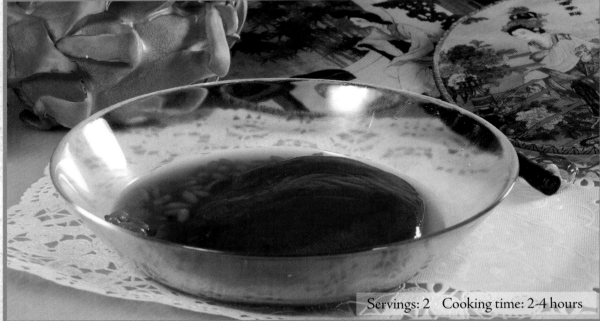

Servings: 2   Cooking time: 2-4 hours

(Liver and wolfberries are shown before cooking to illustrate proportions)

Sugarcane Carrot Tonic

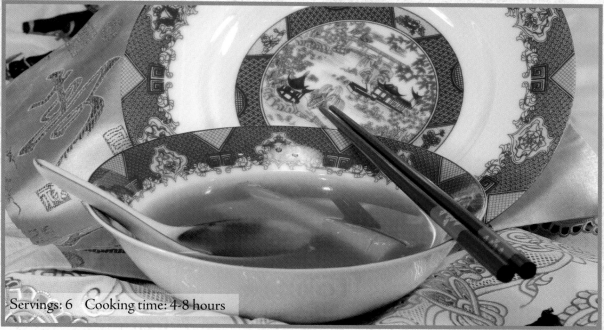

Servings: 6   Cooking time: 4-8 hours

Ingredients

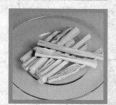

- 1 bag (250 g (8.8 oz.))of "Sugarcane Mix" which contains: dried sugarcane, arrowroot, carrot and imperatae (Rhizoma imperatae)
- Alternatively, 1 bag of fresh sugarcane about 6 links, 15 cm (6 in) long (Both are available at Chinese/Asian supermarkets)
- 3 to 4 large fresh carrots

Optional:
- 1 to 4 cloves of mandarin or tangerine peel may be added to releive coughing
- 125 ml (0.5 cup) black turtle beans
- Salt to taste

Preparation

1. Rinse sugarcane mix or split the fresh sugarcane lengthwise.
2. Wash and slice the carrots.
3. Put all ingredients in pot and add 2.5 liters (10 cups) water, bring to a rapid boil and reduce heat so soup gently simmers for 4 to 8 hours, until very sweet tasting. Discard all solids and enjoy the tonic.

Health Properties

This is a *yun* (moisturizing) tonic commonly used to treat or prevent dryness, dry coughs and constant thirst. It is a great tonic for seasonal dryness. Moisturizing is thought to heal the body and may even slow the aging process.

Salty Arrowroot Paste

Ingredients

- Arrowroot flour (Available at Chinese and Asian supermarkets and some health food stores)

Preparation

1. Mix 15 ml (1 tbsp) of arrowroot flour with about 75 ml (5 tbsp) of cold water to form a slurry.
2. Boil 250ml (1 cup) of water and stir in the arrowroot slurry until it thickens and immediately remove from the heat. Over boiling will turn the paste back into liquid.
3. Add salt.

Health Properties

This is a natural cure for a dry sore throat, as well as for laryngitis. I recommended this to someone who was unable to speak due to a severe case of laryngitis. After consuming two bowls, her laryngitis disappeared the next day.

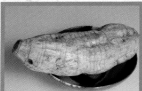
Fresh Arrowroot

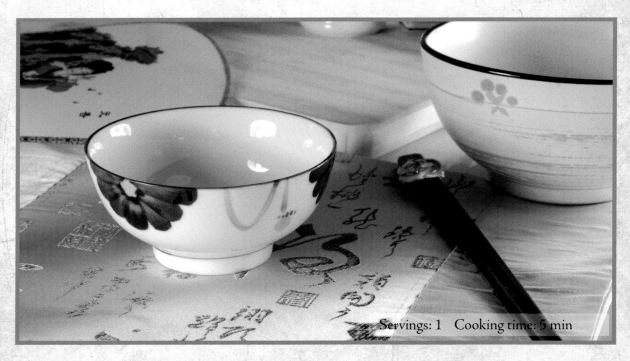

Servings: 1   Cooking time: 5 min

Abalone or Conch Chicken Soup

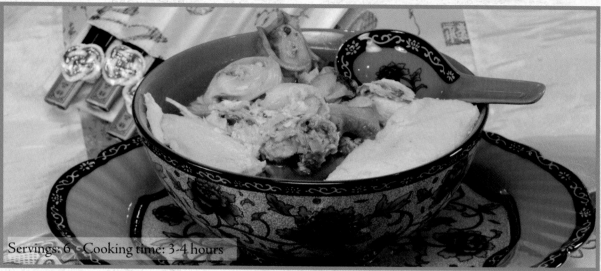

Servings: 6 - Cooking time: 3-4 hours

Ingredients

- 1 kg (2.2 lb) fresh conch or 250ml (1 cup) dried conch or 0.45 kg (1 lb) frozen abalone
- 8 to 15 slices Solomon's Seal (polygonatum)
- 1 piece ginger, about 2.5 cm (1 in) cube (optional)
- 0.9 kg (2 lb) chicken and/or pork

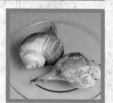

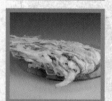

Preparation

1. Blanch the meat and bones.
2. Dried conch must be soaked in warm water for 6 to 24 hours to re-hydrate and to remove any sand. Rinse in cold water and add to the soup at the beginning. Fresh conch must be removed from its shell, by either using a mallet to crush it or by boiling in water and prying it loose. Some Chinese supermarkets will crush the shell for you. The flesh from the conch should be scraped with a sharp knife to remove the black skin layer from its surface. Cut off intestine and discard.
3. Place all ingredients in 3.75 L (15 cups) cold water, adding 5 ml (1 tsp) salt. Bring to a rapid boil for 2 min. Then lower the heat so that the soup just gently simmers. Let the soup simmer for 3 to 4 hours. Skim off all fat. The soup is now ready to serve.

Abalone: If dried slices, use 5 to 8, 3 mm (0.1 in) thick slices, each measuring 50 x 75 mm (2 x 3 in).

If dried whole, abalone must be soaked in cold water for up 24 hours, until softened before use.

If fresh frozen use 0.5 kg (1.1lb), thaw, boil in water for 5 min, rinse in cold water, scrape off the black outer layer, and cut into bite-sized pieces.

If canned, use one 425 g (15 oz) can, slicing the abalone into about 6 mm (0.2 in) thick slices. Add both the abalone and the juice from the can 10 min before serving.

Warning: Abalone is not recommended for anyone with heart problems

Health Properties

This is a tasty seafood soup. This soup is reputably good for the kidneys. It is recommended for strengthening the bladder and controlling urination.

Ching Bo Leung *(Say Mee)* Herbal Soups

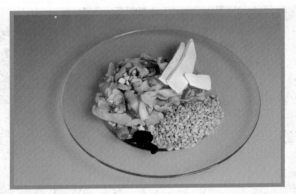

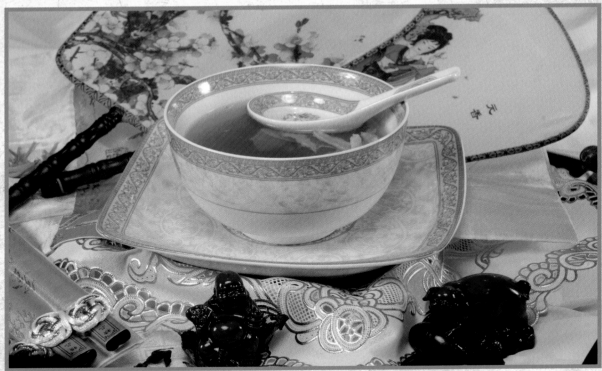

Introduction to Ching Bo Leung Herbal Soups

Chapter 8

Introduction to Ching Bo Leung *(Say Mee)* Herbal Soups

"Sages treated disease by preventing illness before it began. [5]*"*

Ching Bo Leung *(Say Mee)* Soup

Chinese herbalists consider Ching Bo Leung (meaning clearing, valuable, cooling) also known as *Say Mee* to be the quintessential health soup. Its overall effect is to provide both *leung* (cooling) and *yun* (moisturizing) essences to counteract hot bodily imbalances. Additionally it is thought to be a decongestive which reduces phlegm (mucous), relieves chest congestion and eases breathing. Its soothing moisturizing effects aid digestion and elimination and relieve bloated conditions. As well, this soup reputedly aids in breaking down fats and greases, in cleansing the body of mild toxins and in preventing disease.

This soup is my first choice when I do not feel well. Chinese drink this soup in the belief that it is important to provide the body with healing jing/essences to minimize the depletion of the body's own jing/essences, especially during illness. Even if the soup does not cure the illness, drinking a bowl of hot soothing soup will help you feel much better.

Various blends of these herbal health soups are consumed for prevention of illness. A *Ching Bo Leung* prepackage mix is widely available in Chinese/Asian supermarkets and herbal stores. The standard mix has seven ingredients: barley, lotus seeds, longan, lily bulbs, fox nuts, Solomon's seal and dried Chinese yam, which are cooked with pork and/or chicken to make a general purpose health soup. Soup mix ingredients may vary slightly. Other popular blends include *Say Mee* (four herb mix) and *Look Mee* (six herb mix). Although these soups are made from natural food ingredients, those who have doubts or health concerns about possible adverse effects should consider consulting a trained herbalist or doctor before consuming them.

Ching Bo Leung Standard Soup Mix

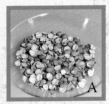

Basic Ingredients

- One prepackaged 140 g (5 oz) Ching Bo Leung mix will make 2 L or 2 qt of soup, unless additional ingredients are added which will proportionally increase the amout of water
- 0.5 kg (1.1 lbs) pork, pork bones and/or chicken
- Alternately, individual ingredients may be used instead of a package as follows:

  A. 15 ml (1 tbsp) lotus seeds
  B. 15 ml (1 tbsp) dried lily bulb
  C. 6 pieces dioscorea (Chinese yam)
  D. 4 to 12 pieces polygonatum (Solomon's seal)
  E. 15 ml (1 tbsp) fox nuts
  F. 30 ml (2 tbsp) pearled barley or popped barley
  G. 15 ml (1 tbsp) dried longan

  Additional optional ingredients may be added as shown below

Warning for People with Food Allergies: This soup contains fox nuts and seeds.

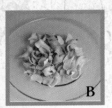

A

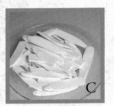

B

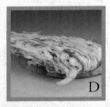

C

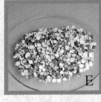

D

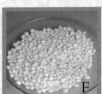

E

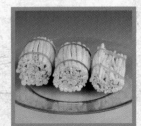

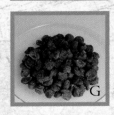

F

G

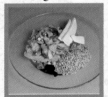

Optional Ingredients

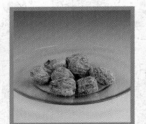

Honey Dates (2 to 4)

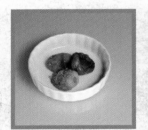

Dried Figs (2 to 4)

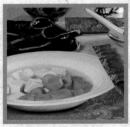

Carrots (2 to 4, sliced)

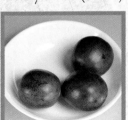

Luo Han Guo
(15ml /1tbsp)

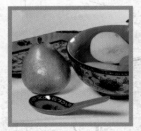

Pear (1 to 2, sliced)

Sand Ginseng / Glehnia
(3 to 8 sticks)

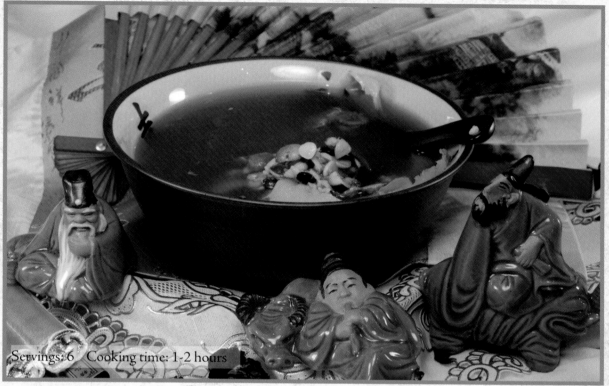

Servings: 6   Cooking time: 1-2 hours

Standard Preparation

This soup can be prepared using just the prepackaged mix or the individual ingredients as shown on the previous page. Additional ingredients are optional and may be added to sweeten the soup and increase its *yun* (moisturizing) effects.

1. Wash the Ching Bo Leung ingredients.
2. Blanch the meat.
3. Place the meat and all ingredients into the pot, adding 3.75 L (15 cups) cold water and salt. The ratio of water to herbal ingredients is about 10 to 1. Bring to a rapid boil for 2 min. Then lower the heat so that the soup just gently simmers.
4. Let the soup simmer for 1 to 2 hours. Skim off grease.

Health Properties

This is a general purpose health soup for healing the entire body. Traditional Chinese consider this soup good for many things. This is the first soup I prepare when I am not feeling well or have an illness. Its overall effect is to provide both cooling and moisturizing essences which can be used to counteract hot bodily imbalances. It acts as a decongestant which reduces phlegm (mucus), relieves chest congestion and eases breathing. Its soothing moisturizing effects aid digestion, promote elimination and relieve bloating. As well, this soup is reported to break down fats and greases and to cleanse the body of mild toxins.

Introduction to Ching Bo Leung Herbal Soups

Four Herb (*Say Mee*) Soup Mix

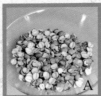

Basic Ingredients
- 0.5 kg (1.1 lb) pork, pork bones, and/or chicken
- A. 45 ml (3 tbsp) lotus seeds
- B. 45 ml (3 tbsp) lily bulbs
- C. 4 to 6 slices dioscorea (Chinese yam)
- D. 45 to 90 ml (3 to 6 tbsp) apricot seeds or almonds

Additional optional ingredients may be added as shown below.

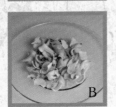

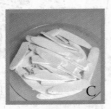

Warning: Raw apricot seeds are a mild poison. Do not use raw apricot seeds or pits. Always buy processed apricot seeds from reputable stores. Do not use excessive amounts of bitter northern apricot pits, as they may be harmful in large quantities. If there are any safety concerns, use regular almonds instead.

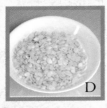

Optional Ingredients

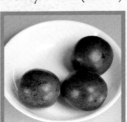

Honey Dates (2 to 4)

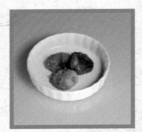

Dried Figs (2 to 4)

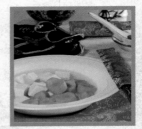

Carrots (2 to 4, sliced)

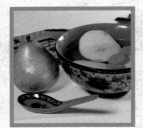

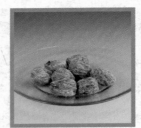

Luo Han Guo (15ml/1tbsp)

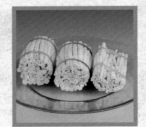

Pear (1 to 2, sliced)

Sand Ginseng/Glehnia (4 to 8 sticks)

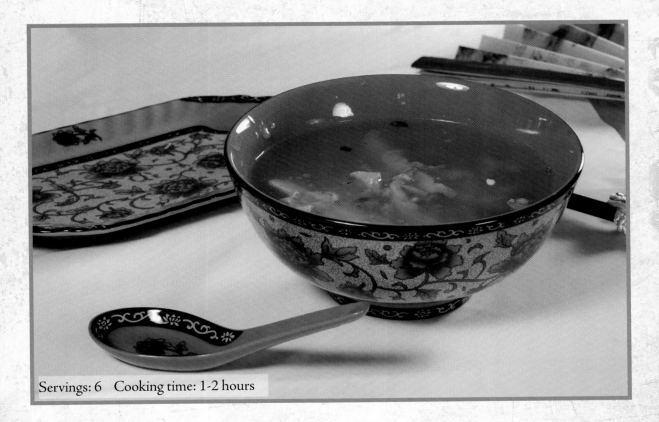

Servings: 6   Cooking time: 1-2 hours

Standard Preparation

1. Wash the Ching Bo Leung ingredients.
2. Blanch the meat.
3. Place the meat and all ingredients into the pot, adding 3.75 L (15 cups) cold water and 5 ml (1 tsp) salt. The ratio of water to herbal ingredients is about 10 to 1.
4. Bring to a rapid boil for 2 min. Then lower the heat so that the soup just gently simmers.
5. Let the soup simmer for 1 to 2 hours. Skim off grease.

Health Properties

This is a versatile soup good for many purposes. It is an everyday soup for prevention. It is often prescribed by herbalists during illness. It is soothing, cleansing and helps restore *leung yit* balance (cold-hot or Yin Yang). If the soup is for illness, determine if there is a *leung* (cold) or a *yit* (hot) illness. If there is white phlegm, or a cold (*leung or yin*) problem use Southern (sweet) apricot pits. If the phlegm is yellow, or there is a hot (*yit hay* or yang) problem use northern (bitter) apricot pits. A half and half blend, may also be used. Almonds may also be used instead of apricot seeds.

Introduction to Ching Bo Leung Herbal Soups

Six Herb (*Look Mee*) Soup Mix

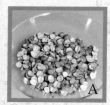

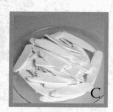

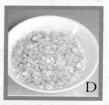

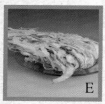

Basic Ingredients

- 0.5 kg (1.1 lb) pork, pork bones, and/or chicken
A. 30 to 45 ml (2 to 3 tbsp) lotus seeds
B. 30 to 45 ml (2 to 3 tbsp) lily bulbs
C. 4 to 6 slices dioscorea (Chinese yam)
D. 30 to 60 ml (2 to 4 tbsp) apricot seeds*
E. 4 to 12 pieces polygonatum (Solomon's Seal)
F. 4 to 8 sticks sand ginseng (glehnia root)

Additional optional ingredients may be added as shown below:

*Warning: Raw apricot seeds can be a mild poison. Do not use raw apricot seeds or pits; buy only processed apricot seeds. Do not use excessive amounts of Northern apricot pits, as they are bitter.

Optional Ingredients

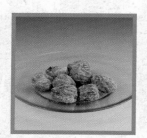

Honey Dates (2-4)

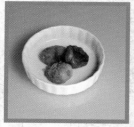

Dried Figs (2-4)

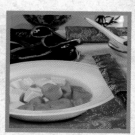

Carrots (2 or 4 sliced)

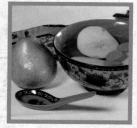

Pear (1 or 2 sliced)

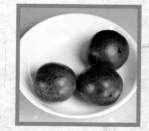

Luo Han Guo 15ml(1tbsp)

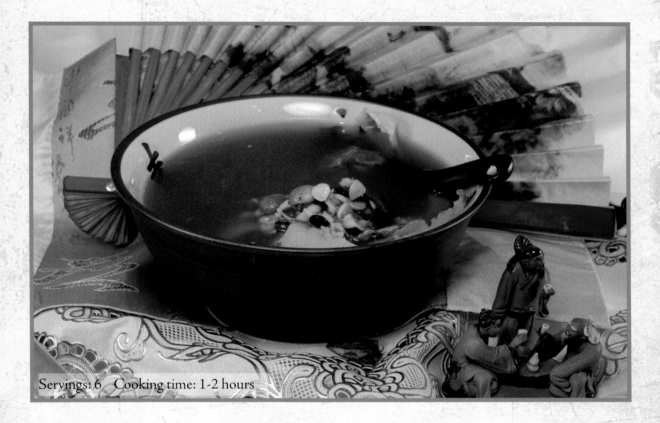

Servings: 6   Cooking time: 1-2 hours

Standard Preparation

1. Wash the Ching Bo Leung ingredients.
2. Blanch the meat.
3. Place the meat and all ingredients into the pot, adding 3.75 L (15 cups) cold water and 5 ml (1 tsp) salt. The ratio of water to herbal ingredients is about 10 to 1. Bring to a rapid boil for 2 min. Then lower the heat so that the soup just gently simmers.
4. Let the soup simmer for 1 to 2 hours. Skim off grease.

Health Properties

This is a versatile soup good for many things. It is an everyday soup for prevention. It is often prescribed by herbalists during illness. It is soothing, cleansing and helps restore *leung yit* balance (cold-hot or Yin Yang). If the soup is for illness, determine if there is a *leung* (cold) or a *yit* (hot) illness. If there is white phlegm, or there is a cold (*leung or Yin*) problem use Southern (*Nam Hung,* sweet) apricot pits. If the phlegm is yellow, it is considered a hot (*yit hay* or *Yang*) problem; use Northern (*Buck Hung,* bitter) apricot pits. A half and half blend, may also be used. Almonds may also be used instead of apricot seeds.

Introduction to Ching Bo Leung Herbal Soups

Wolfberry Pear Herbal Soup

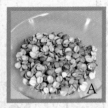

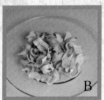

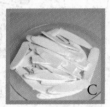

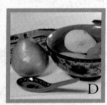

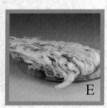

Ingredients

- 0.5 kg (1.1 lb) pork, pork bones, and/or chicken
- A. 30 to 45 ml (2 to 3 tbsp) lotus seed
- B. 30 to 45 ml (2 to 3 tbsp) lily bulbs
- C. 4 to 6 slices dioscorea (Chinese yam)
- D. 1 whole pear, sliced
- E. 5 to 12 pieces polygonatum (Solomon's Seal)
- F. 4 to 8 sticks sand ginseng (glehnia root)
- G. 2 to 4 dried honey dates
- H. 30 to 60 ml (2 to 4 tbsp) dried longan
- I. 30 to 60 ml (2 to 4 tbsp) wolfberry seeds (Guji, Guy Do, Lycium barbarum)
- J. 30 to 60 ml (2 to 4 tbsp) apricot seeds, Chinese almonds*

*Warning: Raw apricot seeds are a mild poison. Do not use raw apricot seeds or pits. Always buy processed apricot pits from reputable stores. Do not use excessive amounts of bitter Northern apricot pits, as they may be harmful in large quantities. If there are any safety concerns, use Chinese almonds or regular almonds instead.

Standard Preparation

1. Wash the Ching Bo Leung ingredients.
2. Blanch the meat.
3. Place the meat and all ingredients into the pot, adding 3.75 L (15 cups) cold water and 5 ml (1 tsp) salt. The ratio of water to herbal ingredients is about 10 to 1. Bring to a rapid boil for 2 min. Then lower the heat so that the soup just gently simmers.
4. Let the soup simmer for 1 to 2 hours. Skim off grease.

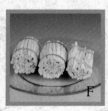

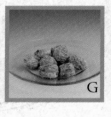

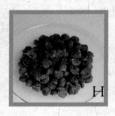

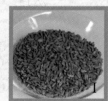

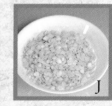

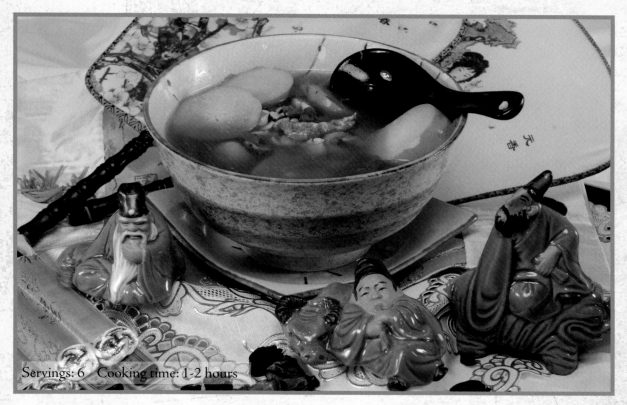

Servings: 6   Cooking time: 1-2 hours

Health Properties

This sweet tasting moisturizing soup is good for cleansing the body, restoring *leung-yit* (cold-hot or Yin Yang) balance and providing valuable healing nutrients. The pear, honey dates and longan are sweet and moisturizing. The sand ginseng, and Solomon's seal are mildly *leung* (cooling or Yin). The dioscorea is neutral and soothing. The wolfberry seeds are good for strengthening the eyes and are reputed to increase sperm count. If the soup is for illness, determine if there is a *leung* (cold) or a *yit* (hot) illness. If there is white phlegm, it is considered a cold (*leung* or Yin) problem; use Southern (*nam hung,* sweet) apricot pits. If the phlegm is yellow, it is considered a hot (*yit hay* or Yang) problem; use Northern (*buck hung,* bitter) apricot pits. A half and half blend, may also be used. Almonds may be also used instead of apricot seeds.

Ching Bo Leung with Winter Melon

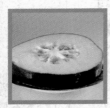

Ingredients

- 1 kg (2.2 lb) winter melon
- Combine with either:
  - 1 prepackaged 140 g (5 oz) Ching Bo Leung mix
  - Four Herb(Say Mee) mix (page 104)
  - Six Herb (Look Mee) mix (page 106)
- 0.5kg (1.1 lb) pork, pork bones or chicken.

Preparation

1. Blanch the meat and bones.
2. Wash the winter melon, remove the pulp and seed and cut into square chunks about 40 mm (1.5 in) per side.
3. Wash Ching Bo Leung ingredients.
4. Place all ingredients in a pot with 3.75 L (15 cups) cold water, adding 5 ml (1 tsp) salt. Bring to a rapid boil for 2 min. Then lower the heat so that the soup just gently simmers. Let the soup simmer for 4 hours.

Note: The winter melon seeds may also be used if desired.

Health Properties

This is a general purpose health soup for cleansing and healing the entire body. Traditional Chinese consider this soup good for many things. It provides both cooling and moisturizing essences to counteract hot bodily imbalances. Its soothing *yun* (moisturizing) effects aid digestion and elimination and relieve bloated conditions. Winter Melon is thought to cleanse the blood, treat skin problems, break down fats and greases and help to cleanse the body of toxins.

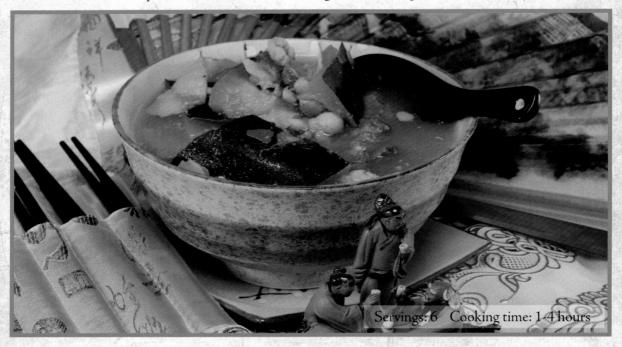

Servings: 6   Cooking time: 1-4 hours

Custom Blending Ching Bo Leung

There was a time when only Chinese herbalists sold Ching Bo Leung ingredients. Today Asian markets and herbal stores sell these ingredients in pre-prepared blended packages and in bulk. Advice on soups and ingredients can be found at Chinese herbal specialty stores. Higher quality ingredients are sold individually or custom blended by herbalists. Knowledgeable consumers often stock ingredients at home and custom blend their Ching Bo Leung.

Since it is only a soup and not medicine, blending to personal taste is often done. We often add carrots to our Ching Bo Leung soup to make it more appealing to those unfamiliar with the taste of this authentic Chinese soup. Other ingredients which may be added are winter melon, apple, brocolli or pear. Carrots and pears are sweet tasting and are moisturizing, good for dryness, sore throats and helping the body heal. Winter melon is *leung* (cooling) and helps the body combat *yit hay* (hot imbalance). It also cleanses the body. It is a good idea to write down your favourite mix, so it can be reproduced at a later date.

See Chapter 4 for an outline of Ching Bo Leung ingredients and what they are good for.

Quick Boiled Chinese Health Soups

Soup Index

	Possible Soup Broths				Page
	chicken	pork	beef	vegetarien	
Watercress Soup	✦	✦	✦	✦	114
Tofu Treasure Soup	✦	✦		✦	115
Fish Maw Seafood Soup	✦	✦		✦	116
Napa with Seaweed (Laver) Soup	✦	✦	✦	✦	117
Seaweed (Laver) Soup	✦	✦	✦	✦	118
Sweet Corn Egg Drop Soup	✦	✦		✦	119
Asparagus Crab Soup	✦	✦		✦	120
Bitter Melon (Gourd) Soup	✦	✦	✦	✦	121
Green Mustard Plant Soup	✦	✦	✦	✦	122
Fuzzy Squash/Opo (*Ded Gar*) Soup	✦	✦	✦	✦	123
Mushrooms and Spinach Soup	✦	✦	✦	✦	124
Chayote Soup	✦	✦	✦	✦	125
Pea Pod Egg Drop Soup	✦	✦	✦	✦	126

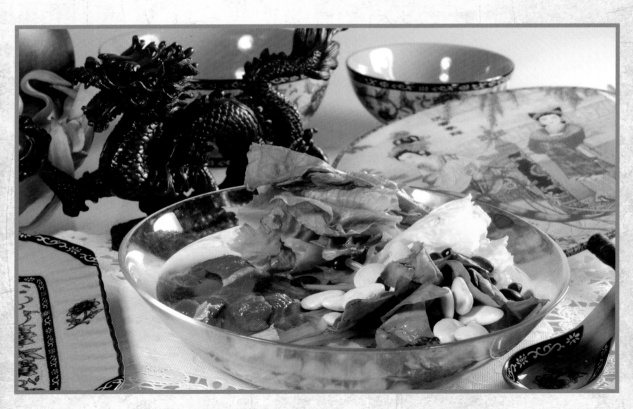

Quick Boiled Chinese Health Soups

Chapter 9

Quick Boiled Chinese Health Soups

Importance of Soup

Chinese take the approach that a healthy soup with meals is important to add protective nutrients into the diet and to counter the strains of modern living. Quick boiled soup is a way of increasing the daily vegetable servings. Chinese believe that soups are a good way to deliver healing vegetable nutrients.

In a world of fast food and long work hours, many people are unable to make soups that take hours to prepare. Chinese often prepare quick boiled soups on weekdays and long boiled soups on weekends.

Quick boiled soups can offer unique health benefits to compliment long boiled soups. Quick boiled soup ingredients are usually consumed because the nutrients have not been fully extracted into the soup broth as in the case with long boiled soups, which require long boiling to access the powerful plant based healing nutrients. Quick boiled soups are generally good for preventing *yit hay* (hot) imbalance, aiding digestion and cleansing, while countering fat and grease. Most of these soups are green and are a good source of chlorophyll. It is a traditional Chinese belief that it is necessary to eat green food each day for good health. They believe that vegetables and beans contain many of the necessary ingredients needed for good health.

Quick boiled soups are usually prepared so that the broth of the finished soup ranges from 70 to 90% of the total soup volume. These soups are usually made with thin slices of meat or dried shrimps that can be cooked in minutes. Alternatively, pre-prepared beef, pork or chicken broth may be used. All of these recipes specify adding salt to taste. It should, however, be noted that pre-prepared soup stocks normally already have sufficient salt.

Watercress Soup

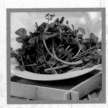

Ingredients

- 2 bundles watercress, 75 mm (3 in) diameter by 100 mm (4 in) long
- 0.5 kg (1.1 lb) Sliced chicken, pork or beef or alternatively use 2 L (2 qt) water or pre-prepared beef, pork, or chicken broth

Preparation

1. Soak and wash the watercress thoroughly several times removing impurities.
2. Slice the chicken, pork or beef into thin slices.
3. Put watercress and meat into pot, add water, bring to a boil and then lower the heat to allow the soup to simmer.
4. Cook for 10 to 20 min. Add salt to taste.

Health Properties

Watercress soup has a minty flavor and is *leung* (cooling). It counterbalances the effect of eating excessive deep fried, greasy or spicy foods. Elderly Chinese who are frail and in ill health sometimes refrain from drinking this soup because they think it is overly tart and *leung* (cold) and may cause them to cough and develop phlegm (mucous). They drink the long boiled version instead. The dark green color of watercress results from its high chlorophyll content, which the Chinese believe to be a basic food substance that protects the body from disease. Watercress is moisturizing and aids digestion. This soup is on the menus of family style Cantonese restaurants.

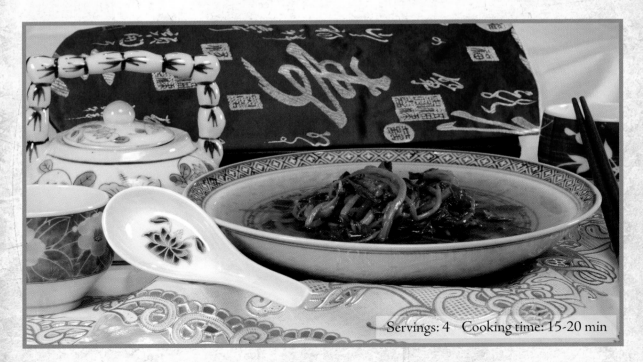

Servings: 4   Cooking time: 15-20 min

Tofu Treasure Soup

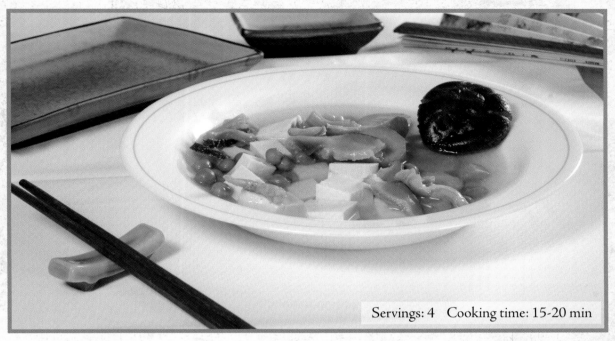

Servings: 4   Cooking time: 15-20 min

Ingredients

- 0.85 kg (1.9 lb) Tofu
- 250 ml (1 cup) fresh or frozen seafood such as shrimp, cuttlefish, scallops, clams, or oysters
- 2 L (2 qt) water or pre-prepared pork or chicken broth
- 45 ml (3 tbsp) fresh or frozen green peas
- 1 large carrot, cleaned and diced
- 1 medium sized fresh tomato, diced
- 125 ml (0.5 cup) fresh or canned corn kernels

Preparation

1. Smell tofu to confirm that it has not gone sour, rinse in cold water
2. Dice the tofu into small pieces. Add all ingredients, except the seafood to the broth. Bring to a low boil and boil for 10 to 15 min. Add the seafood and boil for an additional 5 min. Add salt to taste.
3. Add 15 ml (1 tbsp) starch to 60 ml (0.25 cup) cold water and stir in a small bowl until well mixed. Add to the boiling soup and stir for a few minutes to thicken the soup. Repeat until soup is thickened to desired consistency. If too thick, dilute with boiling water.

Health Properties

This is a tasty soup that has both seafood and vegetable nutrients. Tofu is cooling (*leung*) and helps to offset hot (*yit*) food. Tofu is used to combat water retention and seasonal dryness.

Tofu (bean curd) is cooling, used as an energy tonic, produces fluids, lubricates dryness, detoxicates; affects the spleen, stomach and large intestine. [8]

Fish Maw Seafood Soup

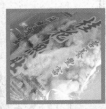

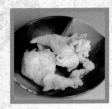

Ingredients

- 50 g (1.8 oz) fried fish maw
- 250 ml (1 cup) fresh seafood such as shrimp, cuttlefish, scallops, clams, or oysters
- 2 L (2 qt) water or pre-prepared pork or chicken broth
- 45 ml (3 tbsp) fresh or frozen green peas
- 1 large carrot, cleaned and diced
- 2 medium size mushrooms sliced or 45 ml (3 tbsp) of pre-sliced mushrooms

Preparation

1. Soak the fish maw in warm water for 20 min until soft and cut into small pieces.
2. Add all ingredients, except the seafood to the broth. Bring to a low boil and boil for 10 to 15 min. Add the seafood and boil for an additional 5 min. Add salt to taste.
3. Add 15 ml (1 tbsp) starch to 60 ml (0.25 cup) cold water and stir in a small bowl until well mixed. Add to the boiling soup and stir for a few minutes to thicken the soup. Repeat until soup is thickened to the desired consistency.

Health Properties

This is a tasty soup that has both seafood and vegetable nutrients.

Fish maw tones the kidneys, increases semen, nourishes tendons, dispenses blood coagulation, reduces swelling and helps to arrest bleeding. [9]

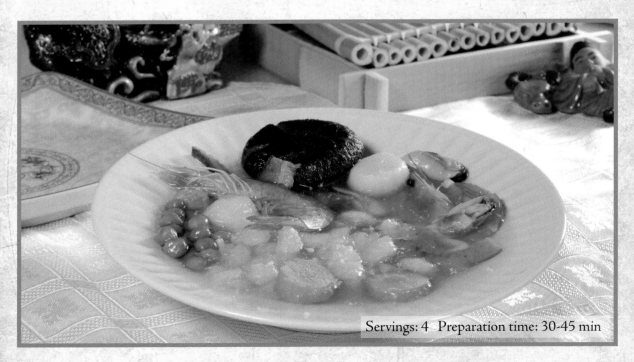

Servings: 4   Preparation time: 30-45 min

Napa with Seaweed (Laver) Soup

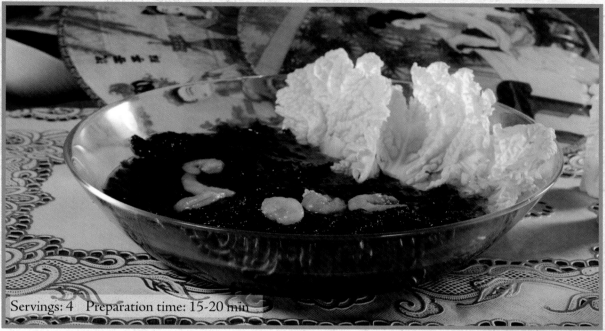

Servings: 4   Preparation time: 15-20 min

Ingredients

- 4 to 8 large napa leaves
- 1/2 to 1 dried seaweed (laver) cake 200 mm (8 in) diameter
- 0.5 kg (1.1 lb) Sliced chicken, pork or beef or alternatively use 2 L (2 qt) water or pre-prepared beef, pork or chicken broth
- 15 to 45 ml (1 to 3 tbsp) dried shrimp (optional)

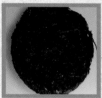

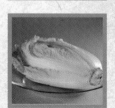

Preparation

1. Wash and cut the napa into bite sized pieces.
2. Soak the seaweed in cold water for 10 min to rehydrate and wash.
3. Add all ingredients to the broth. Bring to a low boil and boil for 5 to 10 min.
4. Add salt to taste before serving.

Health Properties

This soup is cleansing, aids digestion, prevents constipation and promotes elimination. Seaweed is thought to cleanse the stomach and intestines.

Laver removes phlegm from the body, softens up hard swelling in the body, reduces internal heat, promotes urination, strengthens the kidneys, and nourishes the heart. [10]

Seaweed (Laver) Soup

Ingredients

- 1 cake dried seaweed (laver) 200 mm (8 in.) diameter
- 45 ml (3 tbsp) dried shrimp
- 125 ml (0.5 cup) sliced celery (optional)
- 2 L (2 qt) water or pre-prepared pork or chicken broth

Preparation

1. Soak the seaweed in cold water for 10 min.
2. Add all ingredients to 2 L (2 qt) broth. Bring to a low boil and boil for 10 to 20 min. Add salt to taste before serving.

Health Properties

This soup is cleansing, aids in preventing constipation and promotes elimination. Seaweed is thought to cleanse the intestines.

Laver removes phlegm from the body, softens up hard swelling in the body, reduces internal heat, promotes urination, strengthens the kidneys, and nourishes the heart. [10]

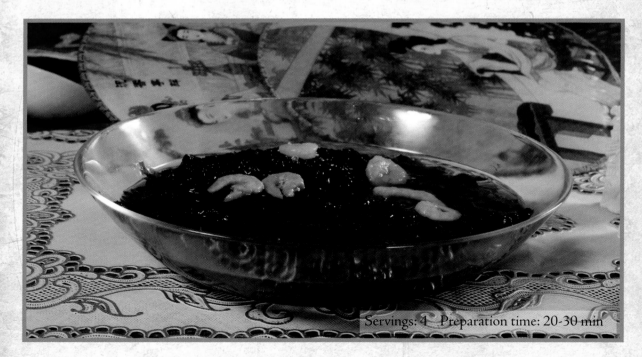

Servings: 4   Preparation time: 20-30 min

Sweet Corn Egg Drop Soup

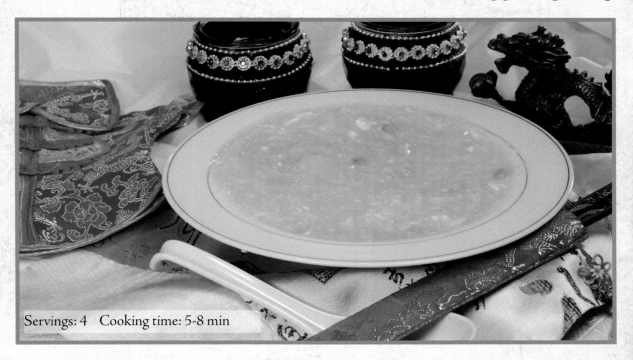

Servings: 4   Cooking time: 5-8 min

Ingredients

- 1 L (1qt) commercial canned cream of corn
- 2 to 4 eggs
- 1 L (1 qt) water or pre-prepared pork or chicken broth

Preparation

1. Bring the water to a boil. Add the cream of corn. Bring back to a boil, stirring occasionally to avoid burning.

2. Crack open the eggs into a bowl and stir to break the yolks. Add the eggs into the boiling soup and stir well. If needed, add salt to taste.

- Optional: Add 15 ml (1 tbsp) starch to 60 ml (0.25 cup) cold water. Stir into small bowl until well mixed, forming a slurry. Add to the soup and stir for a few minutes to thicken it. Repeat until soup is thickened to the desired consistency.

Health Properties

This is a tasty soup and a children's favorite. Corn is thought to assist the **qi** (breathing).

Corn is good for difficult urination, weak heart. Corn is neutral, affects the stomach and large intestine.[11]

Asparagus Crab Soup

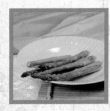

Ingredients

- 0.5 kg (1.1 lb) fresh asparagus

Idea: Use the bottom tough ends of the asparagus for soup

- 426 g (15 oz) (2 cans) prepared crab meat
- 2 L (2 qt) water or pre-prepared broth

Preparation

1. Bring the water to a boil. Add the asparagus and crab meat and bring to a boil. Simmer for 5 to 10 min just until the asparagus is done. Add salt to taste.
2. Add 2 eggs and stir into the boiling soup for egg drop style (optional).

Health Properties

This is *leung* (cooling) soup and promotes digestion.

Asparagus is good for coughs, mucous discharge, swelling, various skin eruptions, shortage of milk secretion after child birth. Crab relieves blood coagulation, cools hot sensations, affects the liver and stomach. [12]

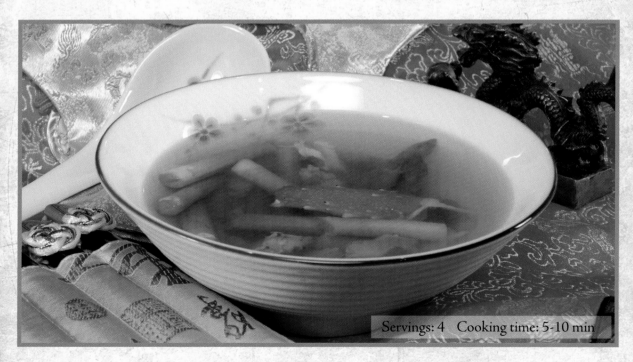

Servings: 4   Cooking time: 5-10 min

Bitter Melon (Gourd) Soup

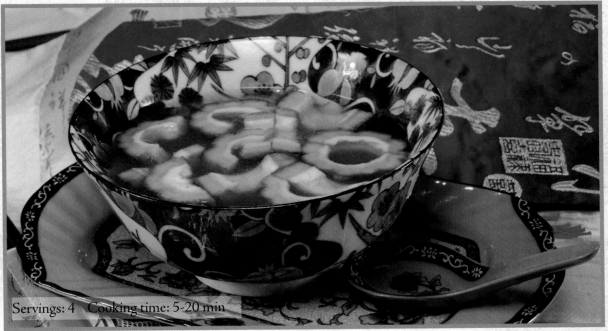

Servings: 4   Cooking time: 5-20 min

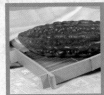

Ingredients

- 0.5 kg (1.1 lb) bitter melon or gourd (*Foo Gar, Leung Gar*)
- 0.25 kg (0.5 lb) lean beef, pork, or chicken with 2 L (2 qt) water or pre-prepared broth
- 5 ml (1 tsp) black bean garlic sauce (optional)
- 30 ml (2 tbsp) small dried shrimps (optional)

Preparation

1. Wash and cut the bitter melon into bite size pieces. The seeds and pulp contain additional healing nutrients and may be included in the soup.
2. Add all ingredients to the broth and bring to a low boil. Continue boiling for 5 to 20 min. Add salt to taste before serving.
3. If the soup is too bitter, add some sugar.

Health Properties

Bitter melon is thought to have many preventive properties against colds and flu. It is a Chinese longevity food and is reputed to be good for the eyes. It has a distinct bitter mint taste and helps to fight off germs. It is *leung* (cooling) and is used to counter *yit hay* (hot) internal energy imbalance. It promotes cleansing, digestion and elimination.

Bitter Melon is cooling, bitter, detoxicates, sharpens the vision, affects the heart, spleen and stomach. [13]

Green Mustard Plant Soup

Ingredients

- 0.5 kg (1.1 lb) *Guy Choy* (Chinese green mustard plant)
- 0.25 kg (0.5 lb) lean beef, pork, or chicken with 2 L (2 qt) water or pre-prepared broth
- 1 piece fresh ginger, 25 mm (1 in) cube

Preparation

1. Wash and cut the mustard plant into bite size pieces. Cut the ginger into smaller pieces.
2. Add all ingredients to the broth and bring to a slow boil. Continue boiling for 5 to 30 min, depending on personal preference. Add salt to taste before serving.

Health Properties

This is a great cleansing soup to counterbalance fat greasy food. The dark green color of the green mustard plant indicates high chlorophyll content, which the Chinese believe helps protect the body from disease. This soup has a pungent taste and promotes digestion. The mustard taste reveals that it is *yit* (warming). Ginger adds more warming properties and is especially good for elderly people and frail people. Good for a *leung* (cold) illness.

Green mustard leaves are warm, good for mucous discharge, cough and chest congestion. It is warming and affects the lungs. Mustard leaves can relieve congestion because it has a warm energy and tastes pungent. [14]

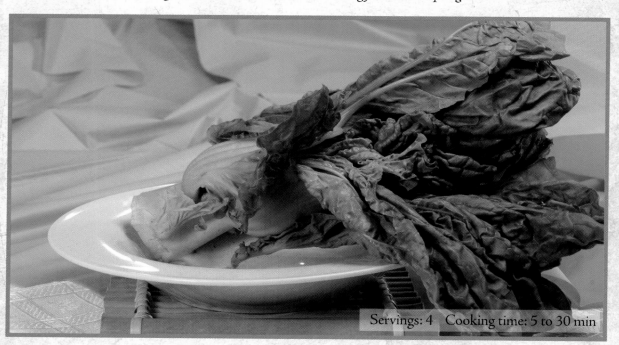

Servings: 4   Cooking time: 5 to 30 min

Fuzzy Squash/Opo (*Ded Gar*) Soup

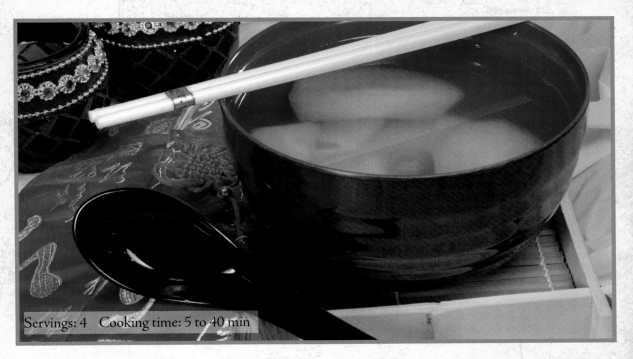

Servings: 4   Cooking time: 5 to 40 min

Ingredients

- 0.75 kg (1.6 lb) *Ded Gar* (Chinese fuzzy squash or opo)
- 0.25 kg (0.5 lb) lean beef, pork, or chicken with 2 L (2 qt) water or pre-prepared broth
- 30 ml (2 tbsp) small dried shrimps (optional)

Ded Gar comes in two different varieties, one with fuzzy skin and one with smooth skin. Either kind can be used in this soup.

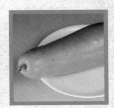

Preparation

1. Wash and cut the squash into bite size pieces. Based on personal preference, the green skin may be removed or may be left in place.
2. Add all ingredients to the broth and bring to a low boil. Continue boiling from 5 to 40 min, depending on preference. When the squash is cooked it becomes translucent. Add salt to taste.

Health Properties

This soup is smooth and clean tasting, aiding digestion and elimination. It is good for counterbalancing the effects of greasy or hot and spicy meals. The dark green skin and icy white interior indicate that it is *leung* (cooling) and effective against *yit hay* (hot) internal energy imbalance.

Squash is sweet, heals inflammation, relieves pain, affects the spleen and stomach.[6]

Mushroom and Spinach Soup

Ingredients

- 0.5 kg (1.1 lb) fresh spinach
- 0.1 kg (0.25 lb) fresh mushrooms or 45 ml (3 tbsp) sliced black shitake mushrooms
- 2 L (2 qt) prepared beef broth (consommé)

Preparation

1. Wash the spinach and cut into bite size pieces. Wash the mushrooms and slice them. The stems may be discarded.
2. Add all ingredients to the broth and bring to a slow boil for 2 to 5 minutes. Add salt.

Health Properties

Spinach contains iron while mushrooms are considered to have many healing properties.

Spinach is good for nose bleed, thirst in diabetics, constipation. It is used as a blood tonic, affects the large and small intestines. [15] *Studies with rats show shitake mushrooms lower blood fat levels. Shitake mushrooms counteract cholesterol. Neutral, sweet, affects the stomach.* [16]

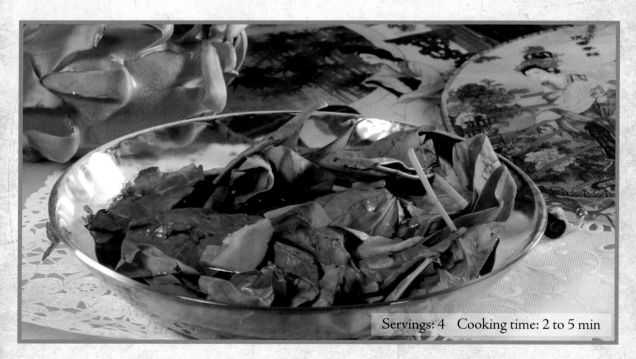

Servings: 4   Cooking time: 2 to 5 min

Chayote Soup

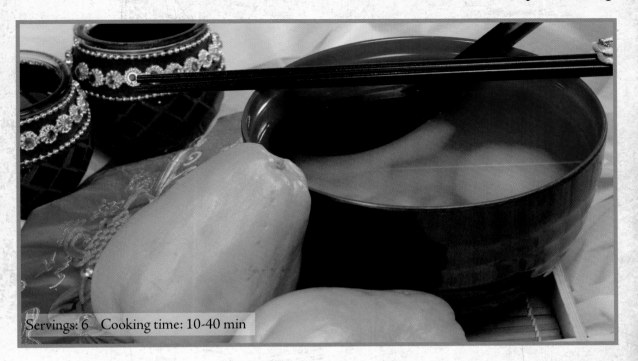

Servings: 6   Cooking time: 10-40 min

Ingredients

- 3 or 4 chayote fruit
- Several thin slices beef, pork or chicken with 2 L (2 qt) water, or prepared beef, pork, or chicken broth
- 30 ml (2 tbsp) small dried shrimps (optional)

Preparation

1. Wash and cut the chayote into bite size pieces. Based on personal preference, the green skin and seeds may be removed or may be left in place.
2. Add all ingredients to the broth and bring to a low boil. Continue boiling for 10 to 40 min, depending on preference. Add salt to taste before serving.

Health Properties

This is a great preventive health soup. It is smooth and clean tasting, promoting the appetite. It is soothing especially when you are not feeling well. It is good for counterbalancing the effects of greasy or spicy meals. The dark green skin and icy white flesh indicate that it is *leung* (cooling) and effective against *yit hay* (hot) internal energy imbalance. Chayote is a popular health food item in many cultures. It is rich in amino acids and vitamin C. Chayote is reputed to have diuretic, cardiovascular and anti-inflammatory properties.

Pea Pod Egg Drop Soup

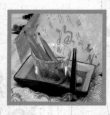

Ingredients

- 0.5 kg (1.1 lb) pea pods (fresh or frozen)
- 2 to 4 eggs
- 2 L (2 qt) water or pre-prepared pork or chicken broth

Preparation

1. Wash the pea pods.
2. Bring water to a boil, add the peas and bring to a slow boil for about 5 min. Add the two eggs and stir well. Add salt.

Health Properties

The pea pods are sweet and moisturizing. The dark green color indicates the high chlorophyll level.

Peas help balance the internal organs, produces body fluids, quench thirst, relieve coughs.[18]

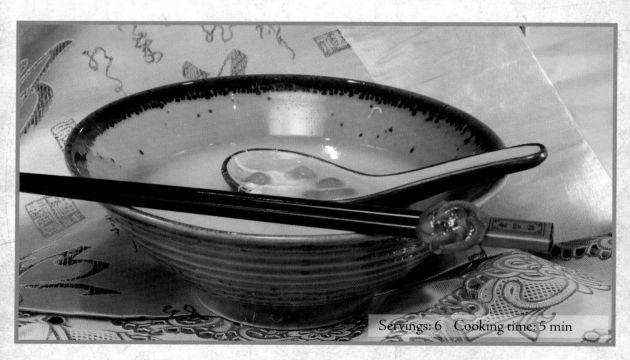

Servings: 6   Cooking time: 5 min

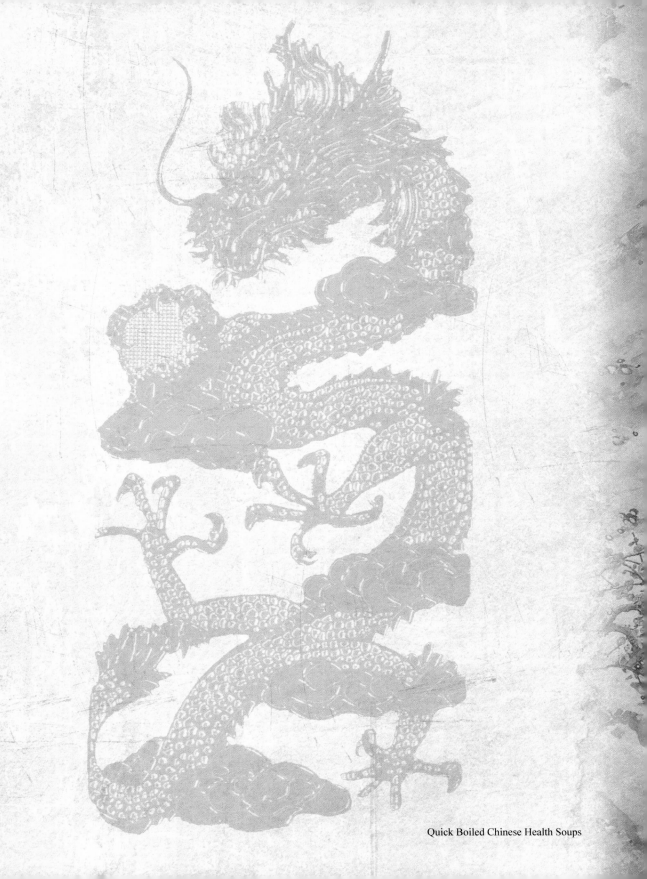

Quick Boiled Chinese Health Soups

Traditional Chinese Congees

Congee Index

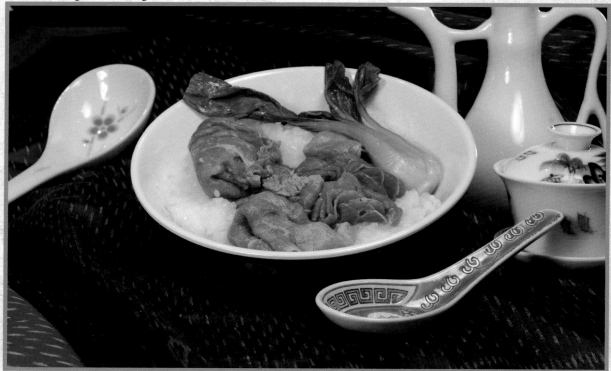

Traditional Chinese Congees

Chapter 10.

Traditional Chinese Congees

This chapter presents recipes for congees (*Jook*, porridge), a rice based soup meal. Congees are often served as a breakfast or lunch item and as a late night meal that is easy to digest. Congees are economical and great for controlling weight, being both low in calories as well as filling. Congees are ideal for breakfast after a large meal the night before. Their high water content helps to flush the system. They are also very good when you are suffering from dryness or dehydration.

Congee Health Properties

One strategy that Chinese herbalists use to fight or prevent illness is to promote urination and bowel movements by drinking plenty of fluids. As well, Western doctors often recommend drinking plenty of fluids when you are cold or sick. Congees are epecially good when you have little or no appetite for solid food. Chinese often serve congees during illness because they are easy to swallow and digest, while providing some nutrients. Congees are considered a comfort food or "soul food" for many Chinese. I can recall times when I was not feeling well, and how a bowl of hot congee warmed my entire body and how its soothing nature made me feel better instantly.

There's a broad range of congees, from the simple, unseasoned rice and water soup to very tasty and exotic congees made with broth and other ingredients. Some people prefer watery congees while others prefer a thicker porridge. Obtaining the desired consistency is simply a matter adding or removing water. The ratio of water to rice is between 1.7 to 2.5 L (7 to 10 cups) water to 250 ml (1 cup) rice. I use a ratio of 2 L (8 cups) water to 250 ml (1 cup) rice. However, the type and variety of rice has to be taken into account. Chinese use long grain or jasmine rice to make congees. The more water used, the more liquid the congee becomes. When the rice kernels are broken, stirring the congee creates a wet paste texture. Restaurants often use a wire beater to break the rice kernels, creating a light creamy style congee. Some prefer a thick congee and eat it as a meal. Others prefer a watery or creamy congee.

The cooking times for the following congees are based upon bringing the soup to an initial boil and then reducing the heat to allow the soup to simmer from 1 to 4 hours.

As an alternative, after initial boiling, the cooking temperature can lowered to 70 °C (160 °F) and the cooking time doubled to 4 to 8 hours. A slow cooker may also be used to make these congees. Start with boiling water and then set the slow cooker for 8 hours at low heat. This is ideal for preparing a winter breakfast.

We often prepare congee just before we go to sleep at night by boiling then lowering the heat to minimum. After 6 to 8 hours, the congee is ready the next morning. Congee can be prepared in 1 to 1.5 hours if cooked uncovered at high temperature. When cooking at high temperature, be careful to avoid spillage, overcooking and possible fire if left unattended.

There are two main methods of preparation. The first is to make plain rice congee and add ingredients such as thin slices of beef, pork, fish fillets, roast duck, barbequed chicken, roast pork or thousand year egg, just before serving. Restaurants often prepare a large pot of thick plain congee and refrigerate it. When congee is ordered, a small amount of hot water is added to a portion of the cold congee. It is heated and the ingredients are added. Raw ingredients are quickly cooked in the boiling congee.

A second method is to add ingredients such as turkey with bones, ham, pork and dried scallops to the rice and water at the start of the cooking process. At home, we always look forward to having turkey congee, every time we have turkey. Turkey bones and leftovers may be frozen for use at a later date; nothing is wasted.

Congees Prepared from Plain Rice Congee

Plain Rice Congee

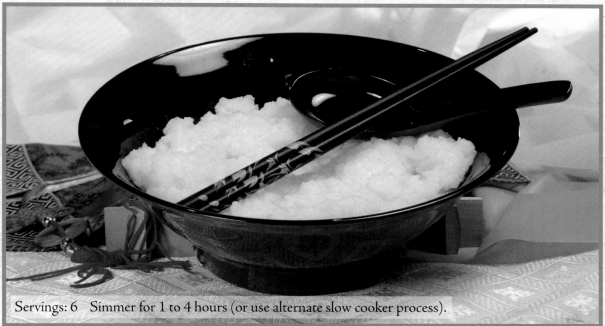

Servings: 6   Simmer for 1 to 4 hours (or use alternate slow cooker process).

Ingredients

Plain rice congee can be served as is, or with meat and vegetables added.

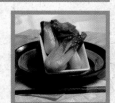

• 250 ml (1 cup) white long grain rice or brown rice

• 2 L (2 qt) cold water

- The water to rice ratio is 8 to 1 but it may be varied depending on the type of rice and personal preference.

Optional Ingredients: depending on personal preference, a number of items may be added to the completed congee, before serving to provide variety. These include: green onions or shallots, peanuts, cashews, flat bean curd, fried dough sticks, rice vinegar, oyster sauce and soya sauce.

Preparation

1. Wash the rice.

2. Add the rice to the water and bring to a boil. Lower the heat and simmer from 1 to 4 hours. Cooking time varies with cooking temperature. Stir when cooked to break the rice kernels, forming a smooth congee. Add salt to taste and any other optional ingredients before serving.

Comment: This can be mixed with Chinese fried noodles, making a tasty soup meal.

Health Properties

Simple, unseasoned congees are used to address colds, fevers and the flu and are considered to provide cleansing to the body. This simple watery soup is also an excellent food for diets as it is both low in calories as well as filling. It helps to flush the system, due to its high water content. This is often the breakfast of choice after a big supper the previous night. As well, vegetables can be added to the boiling congee for a vegetarian congee or it can simply be eaten with a plate of vegetables.

Pork and Thousand Year Egg (Jellied Egg) Congee

Ingredients

- 250 ml (1 cup) white long grain rice
- 2 L (2 qt) cold water
- 0.25 to 0.5 kg (0.55 to 1.1 lb) of lean pork
- 6 thousand year eggs

Optional Ingredients:

- Soya sauce, thin ginger sticks, chopped shallots
- Ham or chicken may be used in place of pork

Preparation

1. Wash the rice and add water to pot and bring to a boil. Lower the heat and simmer from 1 to 4 hours. Cooking time varies with cooking temperature. Stir when almost ready, to break the rice kernels forming a smooth congee. Add salt to taste.

2. Remove the outer layer and shell from each egg. Rinse and slice into pieces about 12 mm (0.5 inch) thick.

3. Cut the lean pork across the grain into short 6 mm (0.25 in) thick slices. Add pork and thousand year egg pieces into the congee and boil for 5 minutes.

Comments

This tasty congee is a favorite at Dim Sum lunches and Chinese noodle houses. It is an excellent food for diets as it is both low in calories as well as filling.

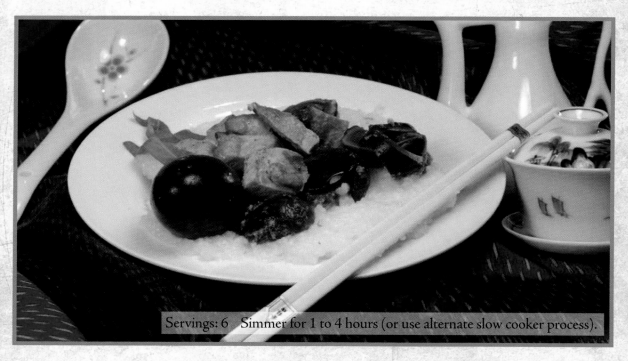

Servings: 6   Simmer for 1 to 4 hours (or use alternate slow cooker process).

Beef Congee

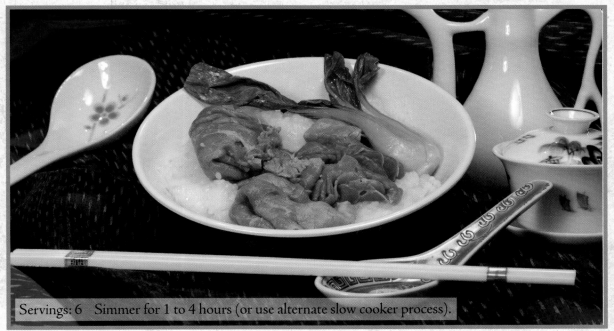

Servings: 6   Simmer for 1 to 4 hours (or use alternate slow cooker process).

Ingredients

- 250 ml (1 cup) white long grain rice
- 2 L (2 qt) cold water
- Thin slices of lean beef such as flank steak

Optional Ingredients:

- Chinese pickled salted turnips, soya sauce, shredded fresh ginger slices, chopped shallots

Preparation

1. Wash the rice, add to water in a pot and bring to a boil. Optionally, add small pieces of pickled salted turnip to give it a deep dried vegetable taste. Lower the heat and simmer from 1 to 4 hours. Cooking time varies with cooking temperature. Stir when done to break the rice kernels. This will form a smooth congee. Add salt to taste and any other optional ingredients.

2. Cut the raw beef across the grain into short 6 mm (0.25 in) thick slices or buy precut thin (fondue) beef. (Beef may be marinated in soya sauce for 0.5 to 2 hours before use). Also, prepare finely shredded fresh ginger (to taste). Place the beef and ginger in the bottom of large soup bowls and spoon the boiling hot congee into the bowls. Stir and serve immediately. The hot congee cooks the beef to medium-rare, very quickly. For those who prefer well cooked beef, let it boil for a few minutes.

Comments

This congee is a staple at Chinese noodle houses. It is a popular breakfast, lunch and snack item. It is also an excellent food for diets as it is both low in calories as well as filling.

Fish (Salmon) Congee

Ingredients
- 250ml (1 cup) white long grain rice
- 2 L (2 qt) cold water
- A piece of your favorite fish fillet

Optional Ingredients:
- Soya sauce, thin sticks of ginger, chopped shallots

Preparation

1. Wash the rice and add to pot of water and bring to a boil. Lower the heat and simmer from 1 to 4 hours. Cooking time varies with cooking temperature. Stir when almost done, to break the rice kernels forming a smooth congee. Add salt to taste.
2. Cut the raw fish into short 6 mm (0.25 in) thick slices. If desired, the fish may be marinated in soya sauce for a few minutes. If desired, prepare finely shredded fresh ginger (to taste). Place the fish and ginger in the bottom of large soup bowls and spoon the boiling hot congee into the bowls. Stir and serve immediately. The hot congee appropriately cooks the fish slices.

Comments

This tasty congee is a good quick meal. It is also an excellent food for diets as it is both low in calories as well as filling. Fish contains omega-3 fatty acids which are beneficial to the heart, brain, digestive system, and joints. It is considered essential to include omega-3 in a diet because it cannot be manufactured by the body.

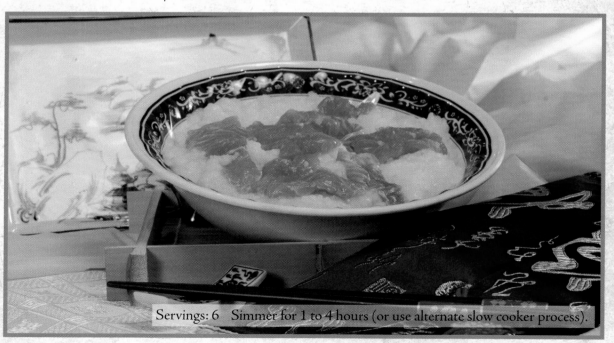

Servings: 6   Simmer for 1 to 4 hours (or use alternate slow cooker process).

Barbequed Duck Congee

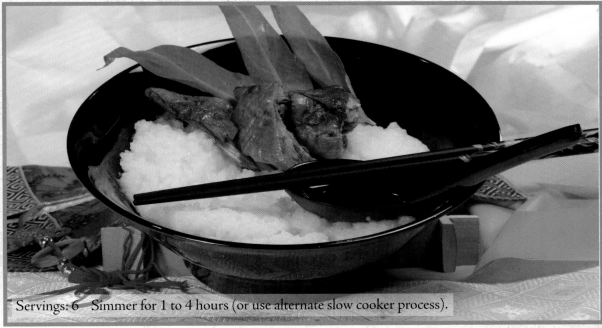

Servings: 6   Simmer for 1 to 4 hours (or use alternate slow cooker process).

Ingredients

- 250ml (1 cup) white long grain rice
- 2 L (2 qt) cold water
- Barbequed duck, chopped into bite size pieces.

Optional Ingredients:

- Soya sauce, thin sticks of ginger, chopped shallots

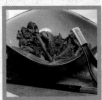

Preparation

1. Wash the rice. Add the rice to the water and bring to a boil. Lower the heat and simmer from 1 to 4 hours. Cooking time varies with cooking temperature. Stir when almost done, to break the rice kernels forming a smooth congee. Add salt to taste.
2. Cut the barbequed duck into bite sized pieces. Add to the boiling congee. Stir and serve immediately.

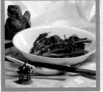

Comments

This tasty congee is popular at Chinese noodle houses. Precooked barbequed duck is available at Asian supermarkets and Chinese roast meat shops. This congee is simple to make. Complete the meal with a plate of Chinese green vegetables such as Chinese broccoli, fried watercress, napa or bok choy.

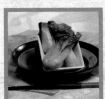

Seafood Congee

Ingredients

- 250ml (1 cup) white long grain rice
- 2 L (2 qt) cold water
- Small portions of the some or all of the following: fresh fish, fresh shrimp, fresh scallops, fresh squid, cuttlefish, oysters, or clams. (Frozen seafood mix is also available at Asian supermarkets)

Optional Ingredients:

- Soya sauce, thin sticks of ginger, chopped shallots, pieces of flat dried bean curd.

Preparation

1. Wash the rice and add to water in a pot and bring to a boil. Lower the heat and simmer from 1 to 4 hours. Cooking time varies with cooking temperature. Stir occasionally to break the rice kernels forming a smooth congee. Add salt to taste.

2. Cut fish, cuttlefish or squid into short 6 mm (0.25 in) thick slices. If desired, these items may be marinated in soya sauce for a few minutes. If desired, add finely shredded fresh ginger (to taste). Remove shells from shrimp. Add all the ingredients to the boiling congee for 2 to 3 minutes. Stir and serve immediately; do not overcook.

Comments

This tasty congee is popular at Chinese noodle houses and is an excellent food for seafood lovers and diets. Seafood contains an array of beneficial nutrients.

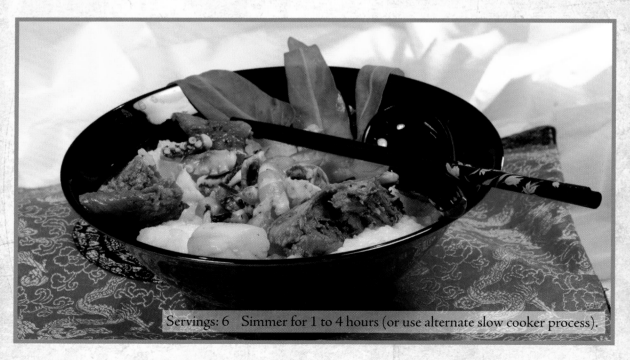

Servings: 6   Simmer for 1 to 4 hours (or use alternate slow cooker process).

Sampan (Seafood and Roast Duck) Congee

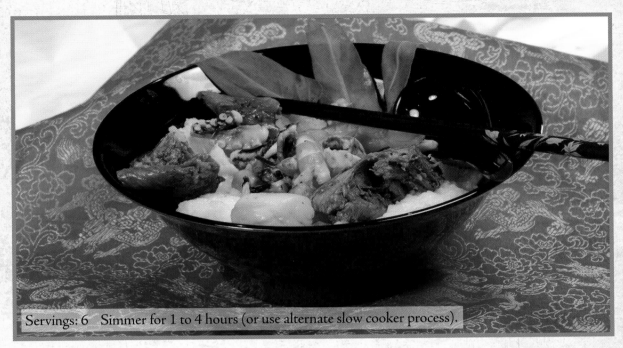

Servings: 6   Simmer for 1 to 4 hours (or use alternate slow cooker process).

Ingredients

- 250ml (1 cup) white long grain rice
- 2 L (2 qt) cold water
- Small portions of some or all of the following: fresh fish, fresh shrimp, fresh scallops, fresh squid or cuttlefish, oysters, clams
- Roast duck, chopped into bite sized pieces

Optional Ingredients:

- Soya sauce, thin sticks of ginger, chopped shallots
- Roasted peanuuts

Preparation

1. Wash the rice and add to water in a pot and bring to a boil. Lower the heat and simmer from 1 to 4 hours. Cooking time varies with cooking temperature. Stir to break the rice kernels forming a smooth congee. Add salt to taste.
2. Cut fish, cuttlefish or squid into short 6 mm (0.25 in) thick slices. If desired, these items may be marinated in soya sauce for a few minutes. If desired, add finely shredded fresh ginger (to taste). Add all the ingredients to the boiling congee for 2 to 3 minutes. Stir and serve immediately; do not overcook.

Comments

This tasty congee is popular at Chinese noodle houses and is an excellent food for diets. Seafood contains an array of beneficial nutrients.

Congees Cooked With Ingredients
Chicken or Turkey Congee

Ingredients

- 250ml (1 cup) white long grain rice
- 2 L (2 qt) cold water
- turkey meat and/or turkey bones
- or chicken meat and bones

Optional Ingredients:

- Soya sauce, thin sticks of ginger, chopped shallots, pieces of flat dried bean curd.

Preparation

1. Wash the rice. Add rice, meat and bones to pot and bring to a boil.
2. Lower the heat and simmer for 1 to 4 hours. Cooking time varies with cooking temperature. Stir to break the rice kernels, forming a smooth congee. Add salt to taste and serve.

Comments

This tasty congee is a favorite during the holidays when turkey is served. Turkey bones and leftovers are used to make a very tasty congee. The amount of meat has a direct bearing upon taste.

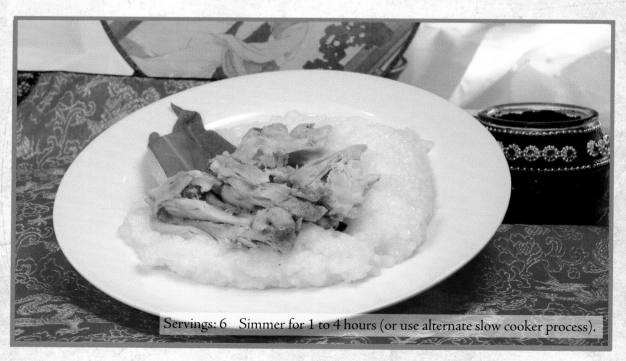

Servings: 6   Simmer for 1 to 4 hours (or use alternate slow cooker process).

Traditional Chinese Congees

Ham Congee

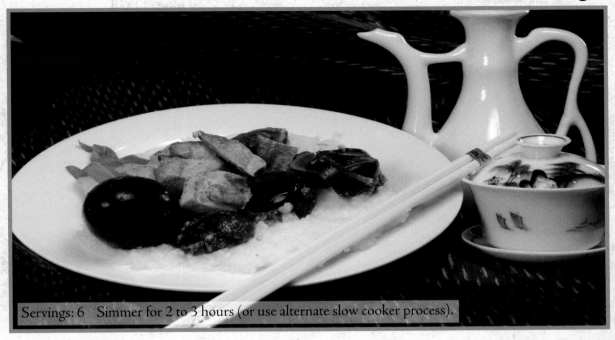

Servings: 6   Simmer for 2 to 3 hours (or use alternate slow cooker process).

Ingredients
- 250ml (1 cup) white long grain rice
- 2 L (2 qt) cold water
- Ham with bone is best, or dinner ham cut into bite size chunks.

Optional Ingredients:
- Thousand year (jellied) egg, soya sauce, thin sticks of ginger, chopped shallots, pieces or sheets of flat dried bean curd.

Preparation
1. Wash rice.
2. Add water to the rice in pot.
3. Cut the prepared dinner ham into 10 mm (0.5 in) cubes. Add the ham and/or ham bone with any optional ingredients to the water and rice and bring to a boil. Lower the heat and simmer for 2 to 3 hours. Stir occasionally to break the rice kernels, forming a smooth congee.

Comments
This congee is ideal during cold weather. It has the taste of ham and is satisfying to the taste buds. It is also an excellent food for diets as it is both low in calories as well as filling. It is a good snack meal. Slices of prepared ham may be added when cooked to make this a hearty meal.

Dried Scallop Congee

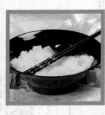

Ingredients

- 250 ml (1 cup) white long grain rice
- 2 L (2 qt) cold water
- 0.5 kg (1.1 lb) chicken, pork, and/or ham, with or without bones.
- 4 to 6 pieces of large 2.5 cm (1 in) dried scallops, or equivalent if smaller.

Preparation

1. Wash rice.
2. Add water to the rice in pot.
3. Soak dried scallops until soft and break into small strands. Cut the meat into bite size pieces. Add scallops, meat and bones to the water and rice and bring to a boil. Lower heat and simmer for 1 to 4 hours. Cooking time varies with cooking temperature. Stir when done to break the rice kernels and form a smooth congee.

Health Properties

This congee is ideal for seafood lovers especially during cold weather. Dried scallops have a deep tasty seafood flavor. It is an excellent food for diets as it is both low in calories as well as filling. It is a good snack meal.

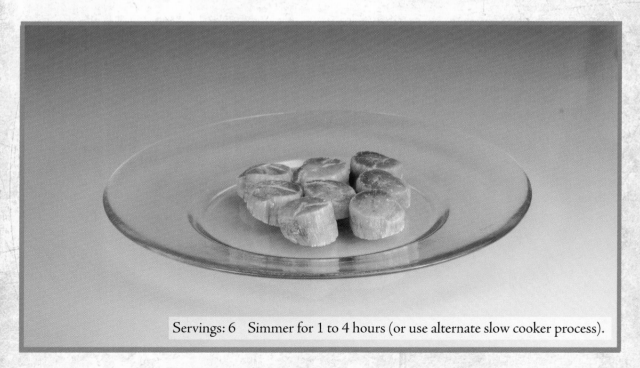

Servings: 6   Simmer for 1 to 4 hours (or use alternate slow cooker process).

Congees Especially for Illness

Winter Melon Congee

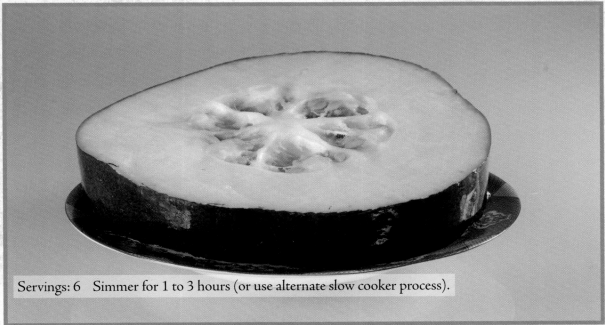

Servings: 6   Simmer for 1 to 3 hours (or use alternate slow cooker process).

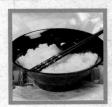

Ingredients

- 250ml (1 cup) white long grain rice
- 2 L (2 qt) cold water
- 0.5 kg (1.1 lb) of winter melon or 250ml (1 cup) of winter melon skin (dried or fresh)

Optional Ingredients:

- Chicken, pork or beef

Preparation

1. Wash rice and add to the water in the pot.
2. Wash and cut winter melon into 25 mm (1 in) cubes. Discard pulp and seeds, keep skin.
3. Add winter melon chunks and any optional ingredients to pot and bring to a boil. Lower the heat and simmer for 1 to 3 hours. Cooking time varies with cooking temperature. Stir when almost done to break the rice kernels, forming a smooth congee.

Health Properties

This bland congee is often served during a *yit hay* (hot illness). It is *leung* (cooling) and cleansing. It is good for skin problems and red rash outbreaks. It promotes urination and bowel movements.

Green Mung Bean Congee

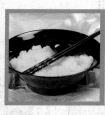

Ingredients
- 250ml (1 cup) white long grain rice
- 2 L (2 qt) cold water
- 125 to 250ml (0.5 to 1 cup) of green mung beans

Optional Ingredients:
- Chicken, pork or beef

Preparation
1. Wash rice and add to the water in the pot.
2. Wash the mung beans and add to pot. Add any optional ingredients and bring to a boil. Lower the heat and simmer for 1 to 4 hours, until the bean kernels are broken. Cooking time varies with cooking temperature. Stir when almost done to break the rice kernels, forming a smooth congee.

Health Properties
This bland specialty congee is often served during a *yit hay* (hot illness). It is *leung* (cooling) and cleansing. It is good for skin problems and red rash outbreaks. It is reputed to be good for helping the body rid itself of *yit doak* (hot toxins). Chinese have long used green mung beans to help rid the body of mild poisoning and toxins. It is not recommended for people who are in poor health or elderly because it is very *leung* (cold) and may cause phlegm (mucous) or coughing. It promotes urination and bowel movements. Mung beans are sweet, soft, easily digested and ideal when ill.

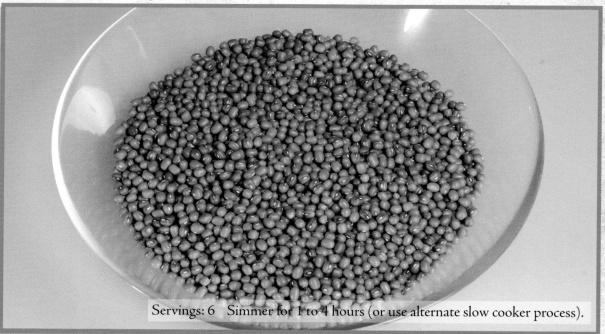

Servings: 6   Simmer for 1 to 4 hours (or use alternate slow cooker process).

Red Mung Bean Congee

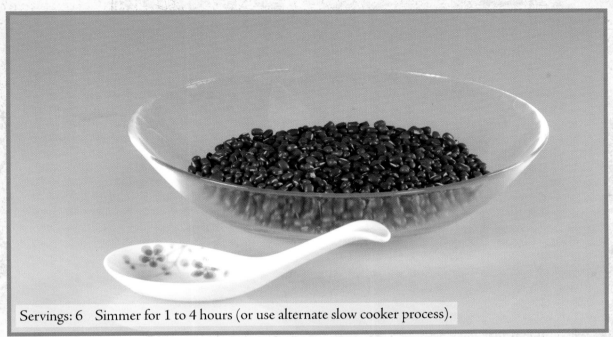

Servings: 6   Simmer for 1 to 4 hours (or use alternate slow cooker process).

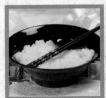

Ingredients

- 250ml (1 cup) white long grain rice
- 2 L (2 qt) cold water
- 125 to 250ml (0.5 to 1 cup) of red mung beans

Optional Ingredients:

- Chicken, pork or beef

Preparation

1. Wash rice and add to the water in the pot.
2. Wash the mung beans and add to pot. Add any optional ingredients and bring to a boil. Lower the heat and simmer for 1 to 4 hours, until the bean kernels are broken. Cooking time varies with cooking temperature. Stir when almost done to break the rice kernels, forming a smooth congee.

Health Properties

Mung beans are sweet, soft, easily digested and ideal when ill. This bland specialty congee is often served during a *leung* (cold) illness. Mung beans are thought to have good healing properties.

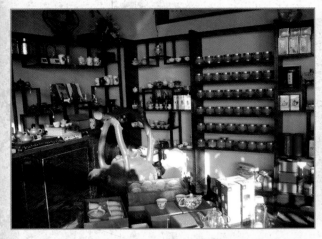
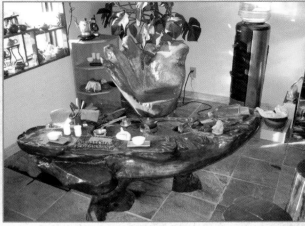
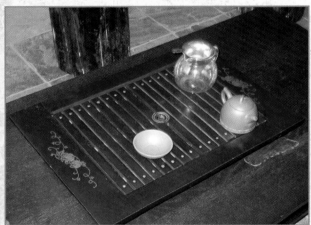
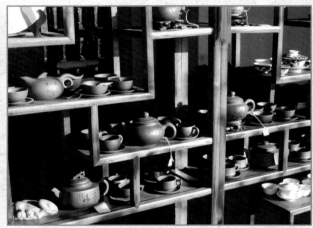

Pictures of tea settings from Cent Tea, Montreal, Quebec

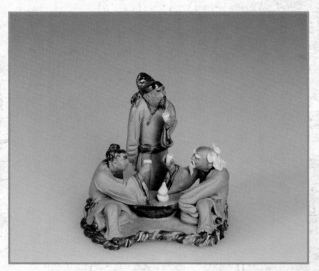

Chapter 11

Chinese Teas

Basics

Many books and articles have been written about the preparation, properties, uses and benefits of Chinese teas. Tea is produced in over 20 provinces in China from tea bushes (***Carmellia Sinensis***). Chinese tea is sold at Chinese or Asian markets and tea stores, which usually carry a large selection. The most expensive grade comes from the top 0.5 % of fine leaves in which only the finest tips or young buds are used. Some of the most expensive Chinese teas are called ***Cha Wong*** (king of tea) and some are infused with high quality American ginseng that gives them a soft pleasant minty taste. However, a good cup of tea can be had on almost any budget, as there are many utility grades which are very good and economical.

There are two basic types of Chinese tea; green (unfermented) tea and dark or black (fermented) tea. The following are variations of green and dark teas:

+ Green tea
+ Oolong (partially fermented) tea
+ Black or dark (fermented) tea
+ Pu-erh or Puer (long fermented) tea
+ Red tea
+ White tea
+ Yellow tea
+ Flower tea

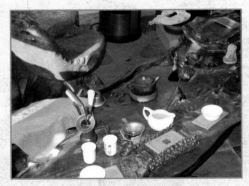

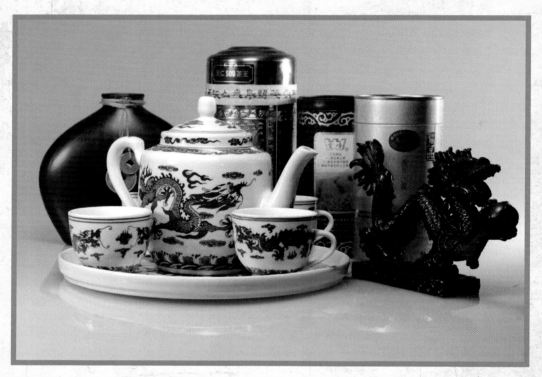

How the Chinese View Tea

Cha (tea) is the most popular beverage amongst the Chinese. The Chinese drink tea with a passion, in the belief that it is essential to good health and longevity. Chinese tea is a pastime, an enjoyment, a cultural heritage and an important health food. At Chinese wedding ceremonies, it is customary for the bride and the groom to serve tea (*Jome Cha*) to the parents and close relatives. Inviting someone for a *Dim Sum* lunch is called *Yum Cha* (to drink tea). At traditional Chinese restaurants, hot tea is served with meals. The most popular types are *Jasmine, Pu-erh, Ti Guan Yin* (dark Oolong), Green tea and *Goak Bo Cha* (*Pu-erh* or Oolong with Chrysanthemum).

Drinking a good cup of Chinese tea can be enjoyable and relaxing. Good teas, especially those infused with American ginseng are excellent thirst quenchers. Tea is prized for its *far ji* (anti- bloating) and grease cutting features. It aids digestion and is often served with meals. The Chinese drink tea to break down grease and to aid digestion. At Chinese restaurants, it is a common practice for waiters to pour hot tea on tables to clean and remove grease. Tea being a diuretic promotes urination and helps cleanse the body of toxins. When not feeling well, the Chinese often drink a pot of hot tea to flush the system.

Some Chinese teas help reduce cholesterol and lower the blood pressure. Tea is believed to slow the aging process, to assist in weight management and to prevent many diseases. Dark fermented teas such as *Pu-erh* or *Ti Guan Yin* (dark Oolong) have a calming effect and are good for settling upset stomachs.

Factors Determining Tea Quality

To some, tea preparation and drinking is a connoisseur's art. A little knowledge of how tea is produced adds to the appreciation of what makes a good cup of tea. Brand names, packaging and what we expect the tea to taste like are what we generally think of when buying tea. However, there are several other important factors that determine quality:

How Was the Tea Picked?

The method of tea picking dictates the selection of tea leaves. How and which tea leaves are picked have a direct bearing upon the taste and price of tea. There are four methods of picking:

- In the imperial method, only the tip or bud is picked. This type of tea was at one time reserved for the emperor and his court.
- In the fine method, the top bud and top two leaves are plucked by hand.
- In the normal method, the top bud and top two leaves are plucked in a less selective matter.
- In the course method, the leaves picked descend down to the fifth or sixth leaf and the leaves are possibly picked by machine. [19]

Where Was the Tea Grown?

Tea is grown in both the high mountains and in lowland areas. Lower priced teas are generally produced in lowland areas, where they are easily picked and mechanical methods can be used. High mountain tea must be picked by hand due to the steep terrain. The climate at high elevations normally produces high quality tea which commands a higher price.

How Was the Tea Processed?

Certain regions which are renowned for their tea may use special processing techniques. Some use secret methods which have been passed down for many generations. The skill and method of production has a bearing upon the final product. Tea is separated and graded in up to eight levels, from super fine down to lower grades. The lower grades may include coarse leaves, twigs and leftovers. Most Chinese are not connoisseurs, but value-minded consumers who normally drink tea that offers good value, so most teas sold at Asian markets are of the good value variety.

Types of Chinese Tea

The following discusses the properties and preparation processes used for the most common Chinese teas.

Green Tea:

Green teas or clear teas (*Look Cha* or *Ching Cha*) are the simplest and most natural of all the teas. Over 50% of China's tea production is green tea. In their preparation, they are naturally dried after picking and then briefly heated or fried to eliminate the grassy fragrance. Green teas are not fermented and retain their green colors as well as natural healing substances like chlorophyll and polyphenols. Green teas are noted to have the highest healing benefits of all teas and are even considered by some to provide anti-cancer, anti-aging and anti-bacterial properties. Green tea has the lowest caffeine content of all the teas. High quality green tea is made from young buds which have a milder aroma and more pleasant taste. Lower grade green teas are less mild; however, some people actually prefer the stronger taste of lower grade tea. Tea experts normally recommend drinking green tea within one-half hour of brewing, after which time it becomes bitter.

Green teas are *leung* (cooling) in nature. Some frail elderly Chinese used to avoid drinking green tea because they felt that it could be excessively *leung* (cooling). However, with today's richer diets and current evidence that green teas have many healing properties, most Chinese now drink green teas regardless of age. Green teas are said to thin the blood and are used to counterbalance and offset the effects of diets rich in meat and fat. Green teas are also rich in Vitamin C.

There are various types of green tea. Gun Powder green is called that because the rolled leaves become small balls that resemble pellets, which upon brewing open up to reveal full leaves. Dragon Well (*Long Jing*) is a variety of green tea that features long leaves. Sencha is a popular Japanese green tea which has a bland mild natural taste. Also popular amongst Japanese is a green tea with fried (popped) rice. It is believed that the rice adds a *yit* (warming) quality to green tea which is *leung* (cooling), making the drink more *leung yit* (cool-hot) neutral and popular amongst the elderly. Sencha and green tea with fried rice are often served with sushi, at Japanese restaurants.

Black (Dark) Tea:

In their preparation, black or dark strong teas (*Hack* or *Nuong Cha*) go through a lengthy withering and drying process, are allowed to ferment for an extended period and are then roasted. The leaves may be withered or nearly completely consumed in the preparation process. Black teas normally have a robust flavor and a mild aroma. They contain the highest caffeine levels of all Chinese teas. Some elderly Chinese prefer to drink back teas as they are considered to be neutral in nature. The fermentation and aging process is considered to add a *yit* (warming) element, rendering black or dark tea as *leung–yit* (cool-hot) neutral. As well, the fermentation and aging process strengthens these teas in their *far ji* (anti-bloating) abilities to combat fat and grease. Black or dark teas are normally used by the Chinese when serving meat or greasy meals to counteract fats and grease, to assist digestion, to break down protein and to prevent bloating.

Oolong Tea:

Oolong (*Woo Long Cha*) tea may be considered as mid-way between green tea and black tea as during its preparation process, it is only "half-fermented". In making Oolong teas, the tea leaves are first spread and withered before undergoing a brief fermentation. They are then fried, rolled and roasted. The leaves of typical Oolong tea may be brownish, grayish, greenish-black or black. Oolong leaves may also be green in the middle and red on their edges as a result of this preparation process. Oolong tea normally has a mild to medium flavor but it may also be quite strong. The fermentation and preparation process is considered to add a *yit* (warming element), rendering oolong teas as *leung–yit* (cool-hot) neutral. As well, these teas effectively combat fat and grease after a heavy meal.

Oolong is one of the most popular teas served at Chinese restaurants and tea houses. It is sold as Oolong or *Ti Kuan Yin* (Iron Goddess). Aged Oolong tea is prized by the Chinese the same way as aged Scotch is prized by many people. Aged Oolong tea becomes milder and acquires a more mature taste. It is not unusual for Chinese shoppers to pick the oldest looking package of Oolong tea, or for people to store it for years before using it. Oolong is a good tea for preventing bloating and settling a bad stomach. It has a calming effect. Oolong tea is often served with greasy meals; to counteract fat and grease, to assist digestion, to break down protein and to prevent bloating.

Pu-erh or Puer Tea:

Pu-erh (*Po Nay Cha*) is a very dark tea that has been fermented in cellars for years, giving it a very strong earthy taste and aroma. It is renowned for its *far ji* (anti-bloating) properties and is very popular with the Chinese for Dim Sum and for dinner. It has a calming effect. It is great for offsetting the effects of a greasy meal and settling a bad stomach. Pu-erh tea comes in various grades. The finer grades made from fine young buds are milder, more fragrant and have a more pleasant taste, while the cheaper grades are harsh, in comparison. Aged high quality Pu-erh tea is prized by the Chinese.

Pu-erh Tea with Chrysanthemum flowers (*Goak Bo Cha*) is a very popular mix, especially at Dim Sum. Pu-erh Chrysanthemum tea is *leung* (cooling) which helps offset greasy *yit hay* (hot imbalance) food, especially at restaurants. Chrysanthemum has a pleasant flowery taste and blends well with the course taste of Pu-erh tea. Pu-erh Chrysanthemum tea is good for treating dryness and sore throats.

Jasmine Tea:

Jasmine tea (*Haong Pin* or *Mood Lay Cha*) is made from green tea with small petals of the jasmine flower. It has a unique smell and comes in several grades. The finer grades made from fine leaves are milder, more fragrant and have a more pleasant taste, while the cheaper grades are harsh, in comparison. Jasmine tea has to be consumed quickly, as it becomes bitter as it stays in the teapot. Jasmine tea is normally served brewed with hot water, but it is also very good with milk and sugar.

Flower Teas:

Flower teas and related scented teas normally use green tea as a base. Dried flowers, such as jasmine and sweet osmanthus are added to the tea at the end of its production process. Flower teas have a light to medium flavor and a medium to strong aroma. Dried tea roses or chrysanthemum may also be added while brewing dark Chinese teas such as Oolong or Pu-erh.

Chrysanthemum Tea:

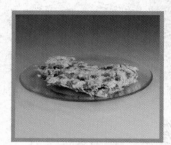

Chrysanthemum tea (**Goak Fa Cha**) is a popular Chinese flower infusion beverage. Chrysanthemum tea is *leung* (cooling) and *yun* (moisturizing) and helps prevent *yit hay* (hot imbalance) and internal dryness. Honey may be added to increase its *yun* (moisturizing) or soothing qualities. Chinese drink chrysanthemum tea for preventive purposes and as a natural treatment/cure against seasonal dryness, sore throats, coughing, fever, flu and colds. It is reputed to have good cleansing properties, aid digestion and elimination. It is a mild beverage good at quenching thirst and may be consumed hot or cold. But it may be more effective as a hot drink when treating an aliment.

Chrysanthemum reduces internal heat, sharpens vision and detoxicates; good for headaches, dizziness, pink eyes and skin eruptions. [20]

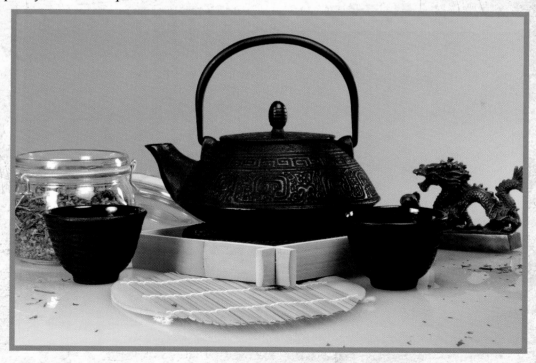

Brewing Chinese Tea

Tea preparation depends largely on personal preference. In some circles, brewing Chinese tea is an art in itself. The water temperature, the ratio of tea to water, the steeping time and even the type of teapot all play an important role in determining the taste and enjoyment of the resulting drink. Some people wash the teapot with hot water just prior to preparation, use expensive clay teapots and serve tea in tiny clay shot glasses. Regardless, the most important factor is the quality of the tea leaves.

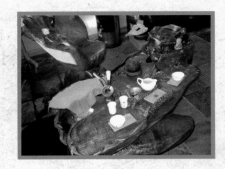

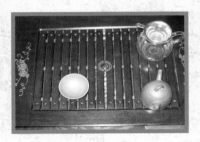

The quick way used by restaurants to make Chinese tea is to simply pour boiling water into a large 0.75 to 1L (3 to 4 cup) teapot containing 7 to 15ml (0.5 to 1 tbsp) tea and let it steep for a few minutes. I personally use boiling water, especially when the water quality is questionable. Depending on how strong you like your tea, vary the quantity of tea leaves and the steeping time to create the desired drink.

Using American Ginseng

American ginseng (*Far Kay Tom*), may be added to Chinese tea to increase its beneficial properties. American ginseng is considered to be *leung* (cooling) to the body. It also helps the body lubricate itself and reduces internal dryness which was considered by the ancient Chinese to be the root cause of many illnesses. Some commercial teas already have American ginseng incorporated into them. As an alternative, you may wish to add American ginseng to your favorite tea. Simply add a few thin slices or a teabag of American ginseng to the teapot before the tea is steeped. It will add a pleasant mint taste and aroma to your favorite tea. American ginseng is sold at Asian herbal stores, markets and tea boutiques. It is available as whole roots, slices and in teabags.

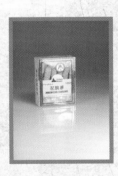

A Trip to a Chinese Tea Boutique

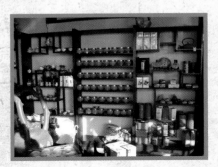

There are Chinese tea boutiques in major cities with large Chinese or Asian populations. They sell mainly Chinese tea. Most are small private stores but there is one major chain (Ten Ren Tea) in North America, which sells only their brands of tea. Tea boutiques carry a wide range of tea, ranging from medium to expensive. They don't usually carry the low priced teas, which are carried at Asian Markets and in some herbal stores.

Chinese Teas

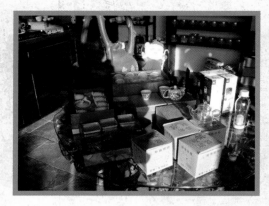 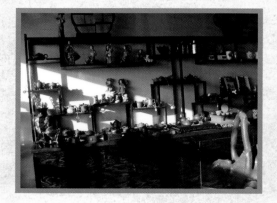

Tea is available in bulk, in cans or packages and as tea bags. The highest quality teas called *Cha Wong* (King of Tea) come in steel cans and are made from the finest Oolong tea, infused with American ginseng and are available as *Ching Cha* (clear green tea) and *Nuong Cha* (dark strong tea). High quality Pu-erh teas made from young buds and well aged are also expensive. These are followed by the fine quality tea and medium quality tea which are available in packages or in bulk. High mountain teas are more expensive than regular or lowland tea. Tea bags are the lowest priced items.

When buying tea you must determine what price you are willing to pay and whether you want *Ching Cha* (clear green tea) or *Nuong Cha* (dark strong) tea, or both. The usual teas available are:

- Oolong, *Ti Kuan Yin* (Iron Goddess) tea
- Pu-erh tea
- Green tea
- Jasmine tea
- Dragon Well (*Long Jing*) tea
- Green tea with osmanthus

Tea boutiques sell American Ginseng in roots, slices and tea bags. They also carry tea roses and chrysanthemum flowers. Some stores will offer tea sampling, if they feel that you are willing to buy some expensive teas. Some stores sell individual cups of tea. Some stores sell teapots.

Herbal Teas

Chinese herbal teas contain or are infused with a variety of herbs, leaves and other natural ingredients. The Chinese use herbal teas as herbal remedies to prevent illness and as a medication during an illness. This is a different approach in that the herbal tea is not a drug but rather a mixture of herbal ingredients that is believed to be able to help the body heal itself.

Chinese herbalists believe that many illnesses are caused by blockages or imbalances in the system and the right herbal ingredient or mixture may help relieve the problem. Traditional Chinese medicine takes into account the *leung-yit* (cold or hot) nature of an illness. Because herbal teas are relatively mild, herbalists generally say, try a little and see if it works; if it doesn't work let's try something else. The three most popular herbal teas are:

Kam Wo Cha

Kam Wo Cha is a *leung* (cooling) herbal tea that is used to prevent/eliminate *yit hay* (hot imbalance), indigestion, hot fever and bloating. *Kam Wo Cha* has herbal extracts infused into the tea leaves. It is available in boxes of ten packages. Each package is brewed by adding hot water in a teapot, just like regular tea.

Lum Tone Cha

Lum Tone Cha (Olive Onion Herbal Tea) is made from perilla leaves, olives, ginger and green onions. *Lum Tone Cha* is a *yit* (hot or warming) tonic, and is used to prevent and resolve *leung* (cold) illnesses, running noses, chills and flu. *Lum Tone Cha* comes in boxes of nine individual packages. This tonic is prepared by simmering for 10 to 30 minutes. Fresh ginger and onion may be added to increase the *yit* (warming) properties, especially when experiencing cool chills.

Wong Lo Kat

Wong Lo Kat herbal tea is a famous brand that has been sold for two hundred years in China and Hong Kong. Herbalist *Wong Lo Kat* came into fame in the 1800's when his herbal mix assisted in curing masses of people during an epidemic in China. *Wong Lo Kat* is popular in Southern China and Hong Kong. Chinese drink it as preventive medicine and during an illness. This tea is thought to be good for helping the body to cleanse, for *gum doak* (to remove toxins), for indigestion as well as for colds, flu and *yit hay* (hot imbalance). Some of the herbalists who taught me habitually prescribe *Wong Lo Kat* for many types of health problems. *Wong Lo Kat* comes in two formats, as herbal tea infused with herbal extracts and in its original format that contains 12 herbal ingredients which must be boiled and simmered for one hour. It is available at some Chinese markets and herbal stores.

While growing up, I knew Jack Wong who was a founder and former president of the Montreal Chinese Hospital. Jack Wong told Professor Chan Kwok Bun, as recorded in "Smoke and Fire- the Chinese in Montreal" [21] , that during the 1918-1919 Spanish flu pandemic, he (Jack Wong) went around the Chinese community with Mr. Xiang, a Chinese herbal doctor ensuring that people were drinking *Wong Lo Kat*. As a result, only two Chinese died amongst a population of three thousand, while the death rate amongst the general population was much larger. He also attributed this feat to the things Chinese eat (and drink), how they grew up in China, their digestive system and so on.

Warning: Herbal tea should be used as a preventive medicine. In the event of a serious cold, flu or other illness, consult a qualified medical doctor. The herbal remedies presented here are not recognized medicines and may or may not be effective. What may assist for one type flu may not work for another. As well, what may assist one person may not work for another.

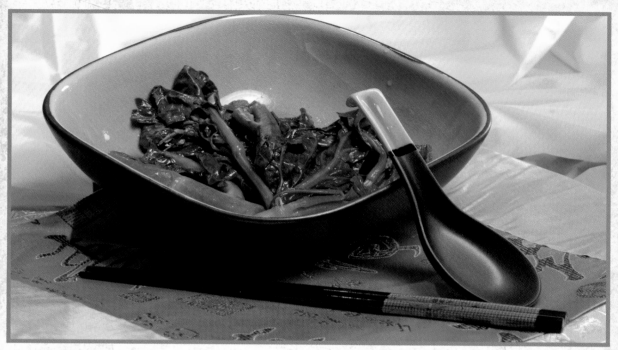

Guy Lan, Chinese Brocolli

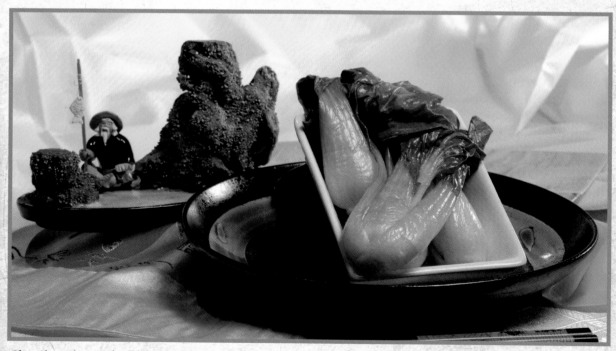

Shanghai Choy, Baby Shanghai Bok Choy

Chinese Vegetables

Chapter 12

Chinese Vegetables

Chinese consider eating dark green vegetables daily essential to good health. Most green vegetables are *leung* (cooling) and provide dietary fibers which promote elimination and cleanse the body. Vegetables provide many plant based nutrients, including chlorophyll the most basic earthly nutrient. There is a great variety of Chinese green vegetables to choose from and cooking is very simple. These are sold at Chinese or Asian supermarkets; seeds to grow these vegetables are also available there.

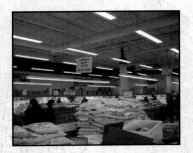

How To Cook Chinese Vegetables

1. Wash and Cut

All vegetables must be washed, some several times until the water is clean and free of dirt. Soak and wash the vegetables in a container or sink to clean and remove dirt.

• The vegetables are then cut into appropriate size. Some ends are tough and are discarded.

• Beans and peas should be nipped at both ends and zip peeled to remove the string strand in the middle.

2. Cooking Methods

Quick and easy ways of cooking Chinese vegetables are:

• Pan or wok fried.

• Steam Fried.

• Quick cooked over boiling water.

• Steamed

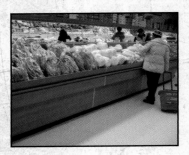

(a) Pan Stir Fried or Wok Fried.

• Heat pan or wok to a high temperature and add sufficient oil to just cover the surface (add more if the preference is for greasy vegetables.)

• Add salt and several cloves of smashed garlic (optional and to taste) into the hot oil, for a short time until the garlic is slightly brown.

• Now add the vegetables into the pan or wok and stir fry until cooked to taste. Vegetables cook very quickly, typically in just a few minutes. Vegetables normally turn darker when cooked. When they are just cooked, they are crispy and crunchy. Those who prefer soft well cooked vegetables should cook them a little longer.

(b) Steam Fried

• Heat pan or wok to a high temperature and add sufficient oil. For those who do not like oil, oil could be omitted.

• Add salt and several cloves of smashed garlic (optional and to taste) into the pan, for a short time until the garlic is slightly brown.

• Now add the vegetables into the pan or wok and stir fry for a minute or two. Then pour a little water, 30 to 60ml (2 to 4 tbsp), into the hot pan or wok and cover. There will be a sizzle from the steam; if done right the hot steam will cook vegetables quickly. Do not add too much water as it will boil the vegetables. Start with a little water and repeat two or three times, if necessary.

(c) Quick Cooked Over Boiling Water

• Boil a pot of water and add a few drops of oil (if desired).

• Add the vegetables into the boiling water and quickly scoop out when the color darkens. Longer cooking will result in more cooked vegetables. Leaves cook very quickly, while hard thick stems take a little longer.

(d) Steamed

• Boil water that is 25mm (1 in) deep in a pot and add a metal steaming stand. Put vegetables in the metal steaming basket, cover the top and let steam for a few minutes until cooked to personal preference.

3. Sauce

Green vegetables can be served with or without sauce or gravy. Oyster sauce or soy sauce may be stirred into the vegetables.

4. Cooking Hard Vegetables

Non leafy vegetables such as chayote, lotus root, *ded gar* (fuzzy squash and opo) are peeled and sliced across, then fried. Dried shrimp may be fried with these, if desired. Stir fried squid or fresh shrimp may be added. Additionally, stir fried pieces of fish, shrimp, and meat such as pork, beef or chicken may be added.

Asparagus is washed and bent until its ends are broken off. Tough ends may be used for soup. Top ends are cut and stir fried. Bitter melon is washed and sliced across. The pulp and seeds are removed then fried with black bean garlic sauce. Sugar may be added if it is too bitter.

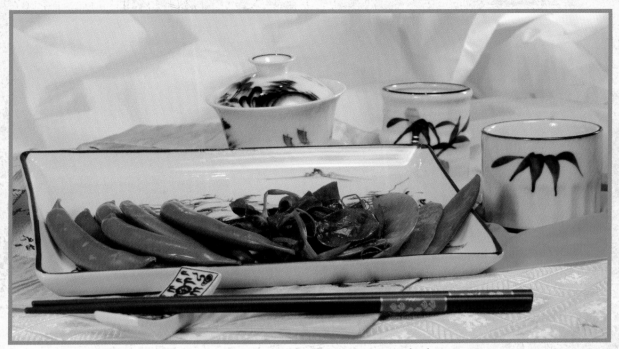

Pea Pods, Snow Pea Leaves, Snow Peas cooked

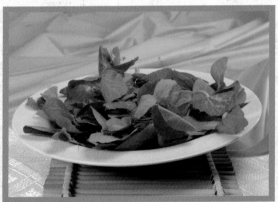

Snow Pea Leaves

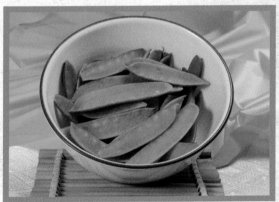

Snow Peas

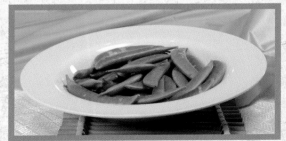

Pea Pods

Chinese Vegetables

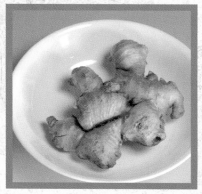

Ginger

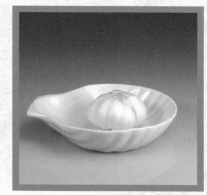

Garlic

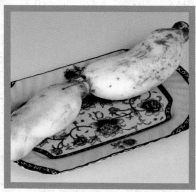

Lotus Root

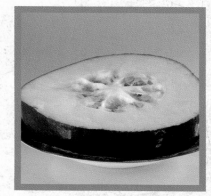

Winter Melon

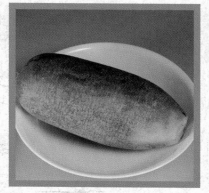

Green Lo Bok

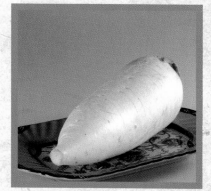

White Lo Bok

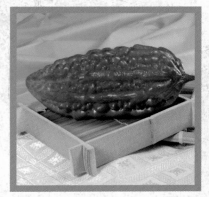

Bitter Melon

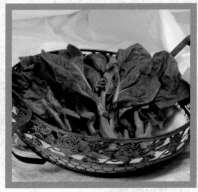

Chinese Broccoli (Guy Lan)

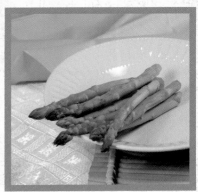

Asparagus

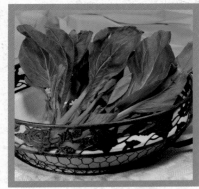

Choy Sum

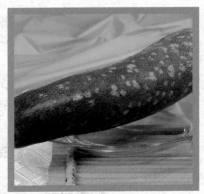

Fuzzy Squash (*Ded Gar*)

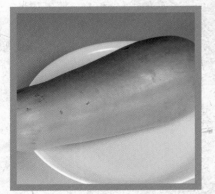

Opo (*Ded Gar*)

Chinese Vegetables

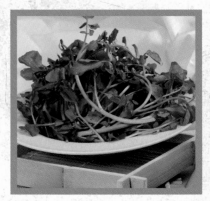

Watercress

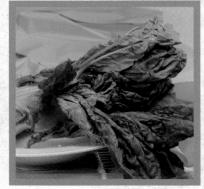

Green Mustard Plant
(Guy Choy)

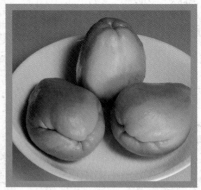

Chayotte

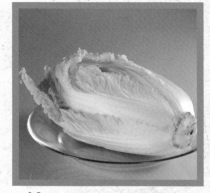

Napa

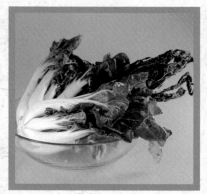

Bok Choy

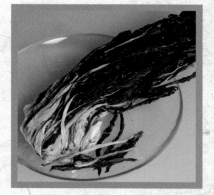

Cole (Dried Bok Choy)

Chinese Vegetables

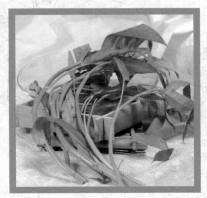

Hon Choy

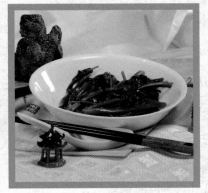

Hon Choy cooked

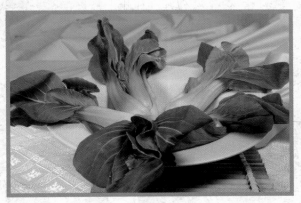

Shanghai Bok Choy

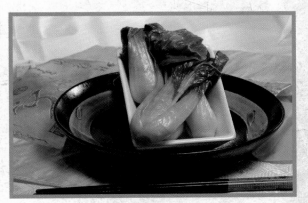

Shanghai Bok Choy cooked

Chinese Vegetables

Conclusion

Chapter 13

Conclusion

In ancient Chinese belief, Yin Yang became the guiding law of the universe when it was formed and had a profound influence on everything that followed. The underlying concept was that the universe was formed by two energies --- Yin and Yang. These two energies then combined to form an additional third energy --- Qi, the life energy associated with animate matter. Everything in the universe then evolved from these three energies, Yin, Yang and Qi. These ancient beliefs have influenced all aspects of Chinese culture, philosophy, health and diet.

Yin Yang's guiding principle is that when everything is in balance, there is peace and harmony. Problems occur when there is imbalance. Traditional Chinese medicine follows this holistic approach that the foundation of health and life is Yin Yang Qi (*Leung Yit Hay*) balance. Healing comes from within. Taking good care of the body involves keeping it clean, active, regulated and provided with appropriate natural nutrients.

While we often focus on physical energy (Yang), the internal energy (Yin) and the animate energy (Qi) are equally important. All three energies must work in harmony to maintain good health. If there is an imbalance in any one of the three, it impacts the other two.

An important objective is to regulate the Yin Yang Qi of the body to maintain appropriate balance. This includes regulating internal dryness by appropriate moisturizing and relying on specific plants and herbs to maintain the internal energy and regulate balance.

Illness may occur when the body is out of balance. The natural way to heal the body and to restore balance is by supplying the appropriate nutrients. Incorporating long boiled health soups is a traditional part of diet and lifestyle and is a key to maintaining good health. Knowing what soups to drink is an important part of traditional Chinese medicine.

Besides maintaining a balance among the three basic energies, mental attitude plays an important part in health. Those who live long and healthy lives also maintain a positive attitude towards life. They live life with a passion and with a sparkle in their eyes. They have a reason for living. They understand that their emotional, psychological and spiritual states have a major impact upon their lives.

Having the right attitude to life, and following an appropriate lifestyle are prerequisites to good health. There is a strong relationship between mental health and physical health which will help avoid bodily imbalances. The ancient Chinese stressed the importance of maintaining a balanced approach to life and emotions. You must remember the good times, when times are bad and remember the bad times when times are good. Taking a centrist approach to life can avoid many health problems.

"They eat food that is often heavy, such as meats and fatty milk and cheese products. Thus they are usually obese people. Externally they are not easily invaded, because they are strong. That is why their illnesses tend to be internal. So treatment for them is herbal." [7]

This was true 5,000 years ago and still true today. Our Western diet is rich and typically boosts our physical energy but it does not support our internal (Yin) and animate (Qi) energies. Our diet often is hot (*yit hay*) and lacks cooling (*leung*) and moisturizing ingredients. Illness often develops from a Yang (hot) imbalance brought on by fattening foods, overeating and lack of exercise. To counter these problems, we must reduce the intake of inappropriate foods --- excessive fats, too many animal products, hot spices and deep fried foods. We must increase our intake of green vegetables, legumes and fruits and supplement our diet with long boiled health soups and teas. Based on Yin Yang this means decreasing the Yang (hot) and increasing the Yin (cool) foods as well as adding neutral moisturizing food and soups. All this is done in moderation to ensure appropriate bodily balance.

The *Yin Yang Qi* strategy takes into account the three principle bodily energies --- internal, external and animate energies and keeps them in balance. As an apprentice, I witnessed herbalist Der Wing analyze health issues by taking the pulse, asking questions regarding health and diet and then recommending a soup to resolve the patient's issues. The most common problems were: *yit hay* (hot imbalance), bloating, energy blockage, internal dryness, improper diet, *leung* illness (cold imbalance) or general energy weakness.

Complex health issues were reduced to simple problems such as bodily imbalance from an improper diet. The solution was to drink an appropriate health soup. From this training I gained expertise with health soups. We normally obtained an answer within a week about the effectiveness of the recommended soup. I quickly came to realize the power of this method of treatment. The body has the ability to heal itself if a condition is addressed at its root cause. Most people neither recognize nor realize what their body is telling them. There is no formal training available that addresses these matters. This method is very safe because using food as a medicine is natural and does not have side effects, unless the patient is allergic to certain food. Dietary problems are the root causes of many chronic health issues. To live a long, healthy life we must develop a positive attitude, know how to address worries, know how to quickly recognize emerging health problems and know how to effectively use food and herbal ingredients to maintain appropriate bodily balance.

As a young apprentice I quickly came to realize the importance of taking care of the body. One of my early lessons occurred when Mr. F. Lee, one of the most prominent Chinese businessmen in Montreal visited my mentor, George Young and revealed that he had developed a major health problem and was told by his doctor that he would soon die. My mentor asked Mr. Lee to tell me his story. Mr. Lee said he had achieved all his objectives of life by obtaining wealth and status within the community but he noted that the one mistake he had made was not taking care of his health. Now it was too late and he must accept the inevitable. He cautioned me that I must not make the same mistake. This lesson had a profound influence upon me. I was later told by my mentor that Mr. Lee died early from high blood pressure due to an imbalanced diet, lack of exercise and obesity.

The road to good health and longevity is to eat simple but healthy foods and not to overeat. Stop eating when you still feel a little hungry. Drink Chinese tea to aid digestion and to counteract fats and grease. Monitor your internal dryness/moisture and your *leung-yit* (cool and hot) internal energy balance and adjust your diet as required. Drink the appropriate soup to provide the required essences, based upon what your body needs. If your body's internal energy is overheated (*yit hay*), cool it down with appropriate soups and drinks. If your body's internal energy is cold and weak, gently warm it with warming (Yang) foods or herbs. If your body is dry, moisten it with soups and drinks that are *yun fay* which moisten the lungs and aid the Qi (breath). Drinking long boiled health soups and teas are critical elements of maintaining bodily balance.

Chronic health problems develop when imbalanced conditions do not receive prompt, appropriate attention. The way to prevent illness is to maintain a good understanding of imbalances and to deal with them as soon as they are noticed. Imbalances may subtly develop and build on themselves causing long term illnesses.

The lungs are the center of our animate energy (Qi). Exercise and deep breathing tone the Qi. In addition moisturizing soups and juices moisten the lungs. Certain soups clear the lungs of phlegm, while others strengthen breathing. Strong breathing greatly influences overall bodily health.

To counterbalance our fattening diets which address physical needs with little consideration for our internal energy needs, eat more dark green vegetables, fruits and legumes. The ancient wisdom is imbedded in long boiled soups and regular consumption must be encouraged. These soups provide cooling and moisturizing (*leung yun jing*)essences required to supplement internal bodily energy as well as to balance and rebuild the body. Drinking tea aids digestion and promotes internal cleansing.

The lessons that I learned as a young apprentice in Chinatown were well taught and became deeply ingrained into my thinking, my approach to life and my diet. I was encouraged to begin this practice early in life, for those who have preserved their jing/essence while young will retain much of it in later life. The wise when hearing of the Tao, try to learn all they can to apply it effectively. For many years, I followed the Yin Yang Qi concept of health without having to give it much thought since it was part of my basic understanding As I got older, my friends began to realize that I was able to retain my health and youthful looks, while they were aging more quickly. They began to comment that my aging process appeared to be much slower than theirs.

When I was in my late 40's, I went for a detailed physical examination and was told that I was in perfect health but resembled someone under 30 years of age. The doctor observed that very seldom does he come across someone like me. He asked for my secret, but I kept it secret because it is so complex to explain. Very few people know how to effectively control their health and aging using the ancient Chinese methods. I am very lucky to have learned these secrets and practices and I hope that this book helps to pass some of this treasured knowledge to its readers.

About the Author

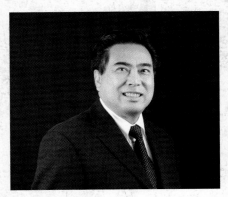

This book on oriental food therapy is not written by a medical doctor. Instead, it is written by a second generation Canadian Chinese wellness expert who learned these skills the traditional way, from the Chinese immigrants in Montreal's Chinatown. He has applied these teachings to his lifestyle for many years. The major health benefits he has received from this way of life are quite apparent. While in his late fifties, with grown children, he still looks, acts and feels like someone aged 30.

Joseph "Gee Ping" Mah is a Montreal-based chartered accountant, who received his formal training at McGill University and gained his business experience at firms such as Deloitte & Touche and Abbott Laboratories, Canada. You must wonder why he has written a book about Chinese soups, congees and specialty foods that promote good bodily health. At the early age of six he apprenticed in a Chinese health food store in Montreal and began his training from the elderly Chinese merchants who were experts in using food to prevent and cure illnesses. In his subsequent business and professional life, he continued to practice the concepts he had learned from his Chinese elders and became a specialist in the preparation of health soups based on his training in traditional Chinese medicine.

It is a known fact that the Canadian ethnic communities continue to preserve the traditions and teachings that were brought to this country by the original immigrants. This heritage includes a rich treasure of knowledge and skills that have long been valued by the Chinese. Current day China has emerged as a prosperous world power through modernization. The Western influence upon Chinese culture, cuisine and thinking is undeniable. But what can the West learn from Chinese? At the top of the list is the knowledge of how to live long and healthy lives without depending on medicine.

In this book, Joe Mah has condensed the ancient wisdom that he learned from his elders and refined through practice, into a modern day wellness book. From it we can all learn the important steps of maintaining good bodily health and staying young through moderation and the selective use of Chinese health soups to keep the body in proper balance. Joe Mah has spent many years learning these skills. Many of his friends have asked him why he is aging so slowly, and, as a result, have asked him to hurry up and write this book.

Glossary: Some Chinese Terms and Concepts

far-ji: To digest without bloating, anti-bloating. To clear blockage in the digestive system.

leung : A "cooling essence" provided by certain soup ingredients and foods (related to yin and complemented by yit). As well, the body may be in a state of *leung* (cold imbalance).

leung-yit concept : When the yin-yang principle is applied to the human body it is known as the *leung-yit* concept. It refers to the Chinese concept of cold and hot internal energy balance. This is the basis of traditional Chinese medicine. For wellness, there must be a balance among bodily forces that is achieved by adopting a lifestyle of moderation, proper diet and appropriate actions. *Leung-yit* imbalance is thought to be the principle cause of many chronic illnesses.

moisturizing (*yun*): Certain food ingredients contain nature essences that help the body lubricate itself, and to promote healing. Moisturizing (*yun*) is used to counteract internal dryness.

principal body energies: The human body contains three principal energies; its internal energy, associated with yin; its physical energy, associated with yang and its animate energy, associated with qi.

qi: The breath or vital force that animates the body.

tao: The absolute principle underlying the universe, combining within itself the principles of Yin and Yang. By extension, Tao also signifies the way, or code of behavior, to achieve harmony with the natural order. The right way to live.

worr: Neutral, neither Yin nor Yang.

worr ping: A neutral and balanced peacefulness.

yang: The active principle of the universe, characterized as bright sun and creative and associated with heaven, heat and light (complemented by Yin). It is regarded as hot or warm energy.

ji: Bloating

yin: The passive principle of the universe, characterized as in the shade or shadow. It is a sustaining energy associated with earth, dark and cold (complemented by Yang).

yun fay: Deep moisturizing of the lungs, which also moisturizes the entire body.

yin-yang principle: Conceptualized more than 5,000 years ago, this principle states that there is a basic balance in nature and that all phenomena can be reduced to an interaction between two opposing forces.

yit: A warming or hot essence provided by certain soup ingredients and foods (related to yang and complemented by leung).

yit-hay: A bodily imbalance caused by excessive of foods with warming, hot essences. Excessive internal heat caused by a hot imbalance.

yun: A "moisturizing essence" provided by certain soup ingredients and foods.

References

1. Ni, Maoshing. The Yellow Emperor's Classic of Medicine. Boston: Shambhala Publications, Inc, 1995. [1]

2. Ni, Maoshing. The Yellow Emperor's Classic of Medicine. Boston: Shambhala Publications, Inc, 1995. p.1 [2]

3. Lao Tzu, Tao Te Ching ,translated by Gia-fu Feng and Jane English. Vintage Books. 1989 [3]

4. Ni, Maoshing. The Yellow Emperor's Classic of Medicine. Boston: Shambhala Publications, Inc, 1995. p.9 [4]

5. Ni, Maoshing. The Yellow Emperor's Classic of Medicine. Boston: Shambhala Publications, Inc, 1995. p.7 [5]

6. Lu, Henry C. Chinese Natural Cures. Black Dog & Leventhal Publishers. [6]

7. Ni, Maoshing. The Yellow Emperor's Classic of Medicine. Boston: Shambhala Publications, Inc, 1995. p.48 [7]

8. Lu, Henry C. Chinese Natural Cures. Black Dog & Leventhal Publishers. p 455. [8]

9. Lu, Henry C. Chinese Natural Cures. Black Dog & Leventhal Publishers. p 462. [9]

10. Lu, Henry C. Chinese Natural Cures. Black Dog & Leventhal Publishers. p 428. [10]

11. Lu, Henry C. Chinese Natural Cures. Black Dog & Leventhal Publishers. p 374. [11]

12. Lu, Henry C. Chinese Natural Cures. Black Dog & Leventhal Publishers. p 418 & 344. [12]

13. Lu, Henry C. Chinese Natural Cures. Black Dog & Leventhal Publishers. p 342. [13]

14. Lu, Henry C. Chinese Natural Cures. Black Dog & Leventhal Publishers. p 428. [14]

15. Lu, Henry C. Chinese Natural Cures. Black Dog & Leventhal Publishers. p 355. [15]

16. Lu, Henry C. Chinese Natural Cures. Black Dog & Leventhal Publishers. p 329. [16]

17. Lu, Henry C. Chinese Natural Cures. Black Dog & Leventhal Publishers. p 403. [17]

18. Lu, Henry C. Chinese Natural Cures. Black Dog & Leventhal Publishers. p 352. [18]

19. Christine, Dattner. The Taste of Tea. Paris: Flammarion, 2006. [19]

20. Lu, Henry C. Chinese Natural Cures. Black Dog & Leventhal Publishers. p 397. [20]

21. Bun, Kwok Chan. Smoke and Fire-The Chinese in Montreal. Chinese University Press. p 117 [21]